Stress Management

A Comprehensive Handbook of
Techniques and Strategies

Jonathan C. Smith, PhD, is a Licensed Clinical Psychologist, Distinguished Professor of Psychology, and founder and Director of the Roosevelt University Stress Institute. He has published numerous articles and 12 books on stress, relaxation, and meditation, and has taught stress management and relaxation to thousands of individuals, corporations, and clinics.

Stress Management

A Comprehensive Handbook of Techniques and Strategies

Jonathan C. Smith, PhD

 Springer Publishing Company

Springer Publishing Company, Inc.
536 Broadway
New York, NY 10012-3955

Acquisitions Editor: Sheri W. Sussman
Production Editor: Pamela Lankas
Cover design by Joanne Honigman

03 04 05 06 / 5 4 3 2

Library of Congress Cataloging-in-Publication Data

Smith, Jonathan C.
    Stress management : a comprehensive handbook of techniques and strategies / Jonathan C. Smith.
        p. cm.
    Includes bibliographical references and index.
    ISBN 0-8261-4947-2
    1. Stress management—Handbooks, manuals, etc. 2. Relaxation—Handbooks, manuals, etc. 3. Health—Handbooks, manuals, etc.
    I. Title.

RA785 .S655 2002
155.9'042—dc21
                                                            2002019468

Printed in the United States of America by Sheridan Press.

9/11/2001

MARK BINGHAM
Passenger on United Airlines Flight 93
who helped thwart the plane's hijackers.

FATHER MYCHAL JUDGE
New York Fire Department Chaplain who ministered
to fallen firefighters at ground zero.
The first officially declared casualty at the site.

RONALD GAMBOA, DAN BRANDHORST,
and their 3-year-old adopted son, DAVID.
Passengers on United Airlines Flight 175.

Contents

Part III: Interpersonal Skills:
Relationships and Stress Management

Preface

I want to thank the many individuals who assisted in writing this book. Alberto Amutio provided considerable assistance in generating exercises, and helped review chapter content. Alberto was also instrumental in the early research that eventually led to the ABC approach to relaxation. I also thank colleague Julie Jenks for her tireless work on collecting data for research on the Smith Irrational Beliefs Inventory. I thank the many students who contributed to the development of all the inventories in this book, including: Eric Chan, Oanh Cao, Demetrios Kouzios, Tracie Dinitz, Rich Piiparinen, and Aaron Karmin.

I thank the 500 Roosevelt University students who used versions of this text for over 5 years as their sole required reading in over a dozen sections of Coping with Stress (a freshman skills course) and Cognitive and Behavioral Coping Skills (a graduate course for master's and doctoral students of clinical and industrial/organizational psychology, counseling, nursing, social work, and rehabilitation). Your experiences and insights prompted many revisions and led to a book I can comfortably claim is thoroughly user-tested.

NOTE

Researchers and licensed professionals who purchase this book may be granted permission to copy and use any of the enclosed inventories for research or clinical purposes. However, inventories must not be altered in any way. Requests to reprint must be submitted to Springer Publishing Company. Any resulting publication must fully cite the present book as the source and acknowledge that permission has been granted for use.

List of Tables and Figures

Tables

Figures

Part I
Stress Basics

1

Stress Competency and the Smith Stress Management Motivations Inventory

We live in an age of threat and uncertainty. Whether it be coping with terrorist attack; war; environmental disaster; economic downturn; or damage to transportation, mail, or medical infrastructures—the need for effective coping is clear and present.

Threats and uncertainties have always been a part of life. All of us have had to deal with such problems as confronting a supervisor over a raise, negotiating an issue with one's spouse, replying to an angry attack, finding a new job, facing an interview or exam, or dealing with the daily din of living. Fortunately, psychology offers us an abundance of techniques and strategies for preventing and managing stress. And the tools for both everyday stress and severe crisis and catastrophe can be found in the same toolbox.

STRESS COMPETENCY

What is stress management? Currently over 100 texts provide a confusing assortment—something of a stress management bazaar. In this bazaar one can find just about anything, including more than few exotic nuts and fruits (see Table 1.1).

The problem with such collections is that they offer few limits as to what constitutes stress management; indeed, every aspect of life that affects how well one deals with threats and uncertainties could be included. Basic skills (relaxation, assertiveness) are confused with situational applications (preparing for an interview, managing extended family, dealing with test anxiety) and health-enhancing behaviors (dancing, eating grapes, petting pets). The result is often a raucous marketplace of

TABLE 1.1   The Stress Management Bazaar

Accupuncture
Aroma therapy
Art therapy
Assertiveness training
Astrology
Ayurvedic therapy
Burnout management
Creativity training
Crystal power
Dating skills training
Dieting
Dream therapy
Exercise
Fasting
Flow training
Forgiveness
Healing touch
Herbal therapy
Hobbies
Hypnosis
Humor therapy
Imagery and visualization
Journal writing
Massage
Meditation
Medications for anxiety
Medications for depression
Mindfulness
Music therapy
Navaho religion
Networking
Nutritional supplements
Pet therapy
Prayer
Problem-solving
Reflexology
Relaxation
Shamanism
Spiritual growth
Substance and alcohol abuse treatment
T'ai Chi
Time management
Urine therapy
Vacations
Vegetarianism
Vitamin therapy
Yoga
Zen

ideas. However, I believe that some forms of stress management are more fundamental than others, and there is an intrinsic order to techniques and strategies available.

I define stress management as a set of skills that enable one to anticipate, prevent, manage, and recover from the wear and tear brought on by perceived threats and coping deficiencies. Such *stress competency skills* focus not only on wear and tear, but on the appraisal of threat, and development of coping resources.

This book organizes the world of stress management into four parts. Part I considers the basics of introductory stress theory. We cover stress competency and basic stress symptoms. Part I concludes with Acute Stress Disorder, an important and timely topic that helps focus and organize our journey through eleven remaining chapters. Once we have a better grasp that effective coping is possible even for severe threat and uncertainty, we can put everyday stress in perspective.

Parts II, III, and IV present a three-part model of stress management that focuses on universal skills, interpersonal applications, and task completion. Specifically: Part II considers universal skills, the four pillars of stress management that are relevant in virtually all stress situations:

- Pillar 1: Relaxing (chapter 4)
- Pillar 2: Planning how to solve the problem (chapter 5)
- Pillar 3: Thinking realistically and productively (chapter 6)
- Pillar 4. Reviewing and rehearsing (chapter 7)

Part 3 considers the application of these basic skills in everyday interpersonal situations. I believe that most stress involves people, and can be managed through some combination of:

- Assertively expressing one's wants as well as thoughts and feelings (chapter 8)
- Listening and responding with empathy (chapter 9)
- Dealing with shyness and social anxiety (chapter 10)
- Resolving conflict and coping with disagreement, anger, and aggression (chapter 11)

Part 4 considers task completion skills for overcoming impediments to applying mastered skills. These include:

- Time management (chapter 12)
- Dealing with procrastination (chapter 13)
- Developing a personal philosophy of life conducive to effective coping (chapter 14)

HOW TO USE THIS BOOK

This book is a manual and textbook for students and health professionals. Relaxation techniques and strategies in chapter 4 can be taught by non-clinicians. Under appropriate supervision, this text can be used in undergraduate courses. In addition, I have taken care to write and organize material in such a way that sections can be given to clients for homework. It is important to note that this is not a book on cognitive-behavior therapy. Therapy textbooks focus on and are organized according to type of psychopathology (with separate chapters for depression, phobias, anxiety disorders, and so on). In contrast, the traditional focus of stress management has been on problems that are less severe. Stress management texts almost universally focus on techniques and strategies.

Suggestions for Client Use

I use the following general format with clients and apply a variety of "didactic" and "practice" tools (see Table 1.2).

1. Orient the client to the limited goals of stress management. "We can't solve everything here, but we can make a start. We have two goals:
   - *Find a Solution.* We will try to zero in on a solvable piece of what is stressful in your life and explore possible solutions.
   - *Learn a Skill.* It may or may not be possible to actually solve the problem we chose to work with. However, selecting a problem gives us an excellent opportunity to learn and practice a stress management skill. Once you have this skill, you may actually use it to solve this problem, or other problems, in the future.

We may achieve one or both of these objectives here. Keep in mind that life is full of problems waiting to solved; we will always have opportunities to learn and try new skills."

2. Empathically listen to the client describe his or her version of the problem. Start with open-ended empathy and move to "problem-solving" and "reality-checking" empathy as described in chapter 9.

3. When the client has thoroughly shared his or her stress concern (including ventilating or "getting it off one's chest"), restate the most important or solvable feature in concrete and specific terms. A clinician might say, "As I understand you, one important part of your problem can be described this way."

4. Suggest as an experiment an appropriate technique or strategy (using the Smith Stress Management Motivations Inventory as a guide). You might say, "I have a stress management strategy I would like to share with you that you might find useful. It may or may not be helpful, but I

TABLE 1.2   Instructional Tools

Various modes of instruction can be used with all of the approaches presented in this book. They include both didactic and practice techniques and strategies:

Didactic Techniques and Strategies

1. *Simple explanation.* Much useful information about stress management can be presented through simple explanation.
2. *Readings.* Information can also be presented by means of selected readings. A client or student can be assigned specific sections or chapters in this book.
3. *Assignment tasks.* Individuals or groups complete a specific pencil-and-paper assignment, and then report their results to each other and the clinician. In completing the assignment task, group or class members engage in discussion.
4. *Journalistic observations.* One nonintrusively observes the behavior of others and attempts to identify behaviors that reflect principles and techniques discussed in this book. One can also observe and note one's own behaviors.
5. *Written homework.* Many exercises in this text are designed to clarify specific constructs (examples: "Find illustrations of assertive and aggressive behavior on television," "Observe and note illustrations of empathy and nonempathy.")
6. *Socratic "questioning."* Using the approach of the ancient Greek philosopher Socrates, one does not present preformulated answers, but offers questions and invites discussion. The goal is to get clients to think for themselves and formulate personal solutions to problems.
7. *Examples.* Illustrations of stress principles as well as effective and ineffective applications of stress management principles enable the client to more readily apply what is learned to him or herself. Illustrations from texts or the clinician's experience can be offered as examples.

Practice Techniques and Strategies

1. *Modeling and role-playing.* Through modeling, a clinician demonstrates the steps of an approach to stress management. This can be done through verbal and written explanation (as in this book), and audio or visual recordings. One can visualize or fantasize the steps required for completing a stress management procedure. In role-playing, the clinician (or other members in a group) actually act out stress management techniques.
2. *Fishbowl.* In a group, two or three members role-play a stress management application while other group members observe and then comment. Comments focus on both strengths and shortcomings of each presentation.
3. *Triads.* Three individuals participate in a stress management role-play exercise. Two actually act out a stress management situation (either an example illustrating mistakes, or an example illustrating useful techniques). The third member sits or stands aside as an observer and offers feedback and possible guiding suggestions during the exercise.
4. *Reverse role-play.* Two individuals role-play a stress situation relevant to one of the players. The situation must itself involve two people (husband and wife, boss and worker, student and teacher, etc.). However, roles are reversed. The individual with the stress problem plays the other person (the stressed worker plays her boss), and the second role-player assumes the role of the stressed individual.

TABLE 1.2   Instructional Tools (*Continued*)

5. *Thought mirror.* Two or three individuals role-play a stress situation. One of them stands behind the individual for whom the situation is relevant and says out loud what he or she assumes the stressed individual is thinking.
6. *Shaping.* A client learns and practices stress management skills in easily learned steps, starting with easy skills, and building to those that are more challenging.
7. *Feedback.* It is important to provide accurate and concrete feedback designed to help improve stress management skills. Positive reinforcement identifies specific behaviors that reflect successful application of techniques. Constructive reinforcement identifies specific behavior deficiencies, including what went wrong and how it can be improved. Feedback can be provided by a clinician, a client, or members of a group.

---

think it's worth a try. If it doesn't work, we can try something else. Would you like to hear it?" If the client agrees, proceed. "Let's try something called [present simple name of technique, for example, deep relaxation, problem-solving, reality-checking, rehearsing, empathic listening, assertiveness training, shyness techniques, anger management, time management, or procrastination management.] This approach is safe and simple, and has been used by many."

5. Explain the technique or strategy, incorporating the "didactic" suggestions in Table 1.2. Give a rationale for how it works, and describe how it is done in simple terms a client can understand. For a complex strategy, give a one-sentence overview, and then describe the first step in greater detail. The following example is for problem-solving. "Here's how one does problem-solving. Basically one defines a problem in the most productive way possible, brainstorms possible solutions, and picks what might work best. The idea is that an entire stress predicament may, for the time being, be too big or complex to solve; but often it is possible to isolate a piece that can be solved. Let's start with your understanding of problems." In this example, problem-solving orientation is considered first. Other components may be presented in following sessions.

6. Review or rehearse the technique, using the "practice" suggestions in Table 1.2.

7. Contract for application. The client specifies when and where they will actually try a specific technique or strategy. Contract for a specific reward a client will give him or herself when application is completed. At the end of the day of application, the client should note in a diary the specifics of what happened, what worked, what did not work, what was learned, and how the technique or strategy might be revised.

8. In the following session, review what has been achieved. Has any problem, or piece of a problem actually improved? Has the client actually acquired any skill? What might be the next step for the client?

In general, I recommend that clinicians take an empathic problem-solving approach, avoiding all of the nonempathic pitfalls described in chapter 9. Techniques are not imposed as "the answer," but gently suggested as experiments. Remember: the clinician is something of a student, learning from the client what does or doesn't work. He or she is a collaborator and consultant, working with a client. Most important, one models the problem-orientation frame of mind described in chapter 5.

Suggestions for Classroom or Workshop Use

Instructors of experiential skill-based courses on coping with stress may find this book a useful instructor resource. Here, I recommend the following:

• I do not cover the entire book, but focus on chapters that reflect class skill deficiencies (indicated by class responses to the Smith Stress Management Motivations Inventory)
• The text focuses primarily on concepts and skills, not examples, illustrations, and case studies. The instructor should provide such supplementary material based on his or her experience tailored to the needs of the class. In addition, examples can be solicited from students.
• I focus no more than half of each class session on lecture material. For the remainder of each class, students form task groups of four to consider selected exercises. Each group reports on the results of their exercise experience, either to the rest of the class or in written homework.

I have had good experience in actually assigning this book as the exclusive text for undergraduate experiential stress management courses. Although it is true that the text frequently addresses "the clinician," I have discovered that the material is sufficiently clear for undergraduate use. In order for such an application to succeed, class goals need to be clearly and appropriately articulated. I find it useful to state two course objectives (1) to provide training in basic stress management skills, and (2) to introduce what might happen in professional stress management. This second goal can be particularly helpful for orienting students who are considering therapy or counseling. In addition, this second orienting goal provides a meaningful context for text references to "the clinician."

This book can of course also be used as a text for courses designed for health professionals (psychologists, counselors, teachers, nurses, social workers, rehabilitation specialists, etc.). Here the entire text is assigned, and students practice teaching techniques to each other or to practice clients outside of class.

Finally, clinicians will find a wealth of workshop ideas in this text. Many chapters, or chapter components (including chapter end exercises) can be readily modified into a workshop format.

THE SMITH STRESS MANAGEMENT
MOTIVATIONS INVENTORY

The present chapter concludes with a simple inventory for assessing and organizing the types of stress management a client or student desires. The Smith Stress Management Motivations Inventory (SSMMI) taps the major skills covered in this text, and was developed and validated by extensive research on over 1,200 college students. Note that scores apply only to a young adult college student population. Check the clinical literature for more recent research on other populations. Generally, research suggests that one can conservatively consider a score higher than "2" on virtually any scale to be a warning sign that a specific approach to stress management may be desired.

To take the inventory, one first answers the questions provided (Table 1.3). Score the inventory using the key in Figure 1.1 (for males) or 1.2 (for females). After obtaining percentile scores from the tables, check the following explanations of high scores (70th percentile or higher). For each scale, I have offered chapters that many of my students and clients have found useful.

Relaxation

High scorers express a need for additional training in relaxation. (Recommended key chapter: 4.) For a more differentiated analysis of relaxation needs, see Smith (1999b).

Solving Problems and Negotiating

Those who score high express a need for basic problem-solving skills as outlined in chapter 5. These include acquiring a productive problem-solving frame of mind, defining a problem, brainstorming options, and selecting a course of action. Empathic listening (chapter 9) is frequently cited as an important problem-solving skill, especially in situations requiring negotiation (key chapter: 5; supplementary chapters: 4, 6, 9, 11).

Managing Time and Dealing with Procrastination

This self-evident dimension refers to skills of organizing one's time and actually committing to and following through a chosen task. Individuals who score high on this dimension are most aware of and troubled by their propensity to procrastinate, suggesting that self-reported procrastination can serve as an initial focus in intervention (key chapters: 12, 13; supplementary chapter: 14)

TABLE 1.3 The Smith Stress Management Motivations Inventory (SSMMI)

The following items describe different stress management skills many people find useful. What stress management skills would you like to learn or perfect? Please rate **each item** in the blanks to the left. Use this key

I would like to learn or perfect this skill . . .

1 = Not at All (I do not lack or need this skill)
2 = A Little
3 = Moderately
4 = Very Much

① ② ③ ④   1.   How to bargain effectively in an adult way.
① ② ③ ④   2.   How to stop obsessive thinking.
① ② ③ ④   3.   How to feel less anxious and nervous.
① ② ③ ④   4.   How to calm my heartbeat when it is too fast, hard, or irregular.
① ② ③ ④   5.   How to use relaxation to reduce physical pain.
① ② ③ ④   6.   How to say no to requests from others.
① ② ③ ④   7.   How to prevent and recover from a backache.
① ② ③ ④   8.   How to practice a relaxation technique that will help me feel more at ease and peaceful.
① ② ③ ④   9.   How to settle my differences with others so that we both come out ahead.
① ② ③ ④   10.   How to be less anxious or nervous when being watched during sports (or workouts).
① ② ③ ④   11.   How to approach someone I would like to meet and "break the ice" to start a conversation.
① ② ③ ④   12.   How to say "stop" when thinking about a problem isn't getting me anywhere.
① ② ③ ④   13.   How to respond more constructively when my anger is provoked.
① ② ③ ④   14.   How to soothe my nervous stomach.
① ② ③ ④   15.   How to feel less depressed.
① ② ③ ④   16.   How to be less anxious or nervous about making a mistake in front of others.
① ② ③ ④   17.   How to avoid putting off doing things until it is too late.
① ② ③ ④   18.   How to develop strategies for managing my physical pain.
① ② ③ ④   19.   How to tell someone their behavior bothers me.
① ② ③ ④   20.   How to prevent and recover from a headache.
① ② ③ ④   21.   How to figure out ahead of time which choices might and might not work.
① ② ③ ④   22.   How to deal with my own anger and aggressiveness more effectively.
① ② ③ ④   23.   How to deal with loss of appetite.
① ② ③ ④   24.   How to stop worrying when it's time to do something else.
① ② ③ ④   25.   How to renew or maintain contact with someone I've already met or know.
① ② ③ ④   26.   How to develop thinking patterns that reduce physical pain.

TABLE 1.3   The Smith Stress Management Motivations Inventory (SSMMI) (*Continued*)

① ② ③ ④	27.	How to listen in such a way that builds cooperation and friendship.
① ② ③ ④	28.	How to be less anxious or nervous when eating or drinking in front of others.
① ② ③ ④	29.	How to say what's on my mind and be taken seriously.
① ② ③ ④	30.	How to deal with my procrastination.
① ② ③ ④	31.	How to practice a relaxation technique that will help me feel more happy and joyful.
① ② ③ ④	32.	How to avoid and reduce tension in my shoulders, neck, or back.
① ② ③ ④	33.	How to "cool off" and keep my anger from rising to dangerous levels.
① ② ③ ④	34.	How to deal with problem perspiration or feeling too warm.
① ② ③ ④	35.	How to find good places and situations for meeting people.
① ② ③ ④	36.	How to decide what course of action will do the greatest good.
① ② ③ ④	37.	How to respond when others verbally attack me.
① ② ③ ④	38.	How to be less tense or self-conscious when doing things in public (where others can see me).
① ② ③ ④	39.	How to identify useful early warning signs for preventing physical pain attacks.
① ② ③ ④	40.	How to stop thinking when I've thought about a problem enough.
① ② ③ ④	41.	How to be less fearful and apprehensive.
① ② ③ ④	42.	How to increase my ability to think of useful alternatives.
① ② ③ ④	43.	How to avoid "blowing up" with destructive anger.
① ② ③ ④	44.	How to effectively treat dryness in my mouth.
① ② ③ ④	45.	How to feel less distressed (discouraged or sad).
① ② ③ ④	46.	How to stop putting off responsibilities.
① ② ③ ④	47.	How to think of new solutions to old problems.
① ② ③ ④	48.	How to have less muscle tension (muscles tight, tense, or clenched up; furrowed brow, tightened fist, clenched jaw).
① ② ③ ④	49.	How to keep a conversation going after I've met someone.
① ② ③ ④	50.	How to reduce the tendency for my eyes to water or get teary.
① ② ③ ④	51.	How to practice a relaxation exercise that will help me feel more strengthened, energized, and aware.
① ② ③ ④	52.	How to stop jumping to conclusions about how bad things are.
① ② ③ ④	53.	How to weigh the costs and benefits of actions before I do them.
① ② ③ ④	54.	How to effectively make requests.
① ② ③ ④	55.	How to manage my time more effectively.
① ② ③ ④	56.	How to figure out when is the best time to act on a problem.
① ② ③ ④	57.	How to stop avoiding what I should be doing.
① ② ③ ④	58.	How to breathe in a way that is less tense, hurried, shallow, or uneven.
① ② ③ ④	59.	How to be less anxious or nervous when speaking or performing in front of others.

SCALES (Scoring Key)

INSTRUCTIONS: Add items in parentheses. Then divide the sum by the number to the right of the "/" mark. Thus, to obtain one's score for the "Managing Anxiety" scale, first add the responses to items 3 and 41. Then divide this by 2. Finally, find the appropriate match in the "ESTIMATED PERCENTILES" table to the right.

ESTIMATED PERCENTILES

For each scale, find percentile score below that most closely matches SCOREBOX score. If there is no exact match, select closest lower percentile score. Percentile means "Score is higher than X% of sample."

SCALES (Scoring Key)	M (sd)	SCOREBOX	10	20	30	40	50	60	70	80	90	100
Relaxation (8 + 31 + 51) / 3	2.35 (.77)		1.22	1.67	2.00	2.11	2.33	2.55	2.77	3.00	3.44	4

SMITH STRESS MANAGEMENT MOTIVATIONS INVENTORY

SCALES (Scoring Key)	M (sd)	10	20	30	40	50	60	70	80	90	100
Solving Problems and Negotiating (1 + 9 + 21 + 27 + 36 + 42 + 47 + 53 + 56) / 9	2.68 (.85)	1.4	2	2.2	2.4	2.8	3	3.2	3.4	3.8	4
Managing Time and Dealing with Procrastination (17 + 30 + 46 + 55 + 57) / 5	2.34 (.82)	1.2	1.6	1.8	2	2.3	2.6	2.8	3	3.6	4
Managing Worry (2 + 12 + 24 + 40 + 52) / 5	2.73 (.94)	1.25	1.75	2.25	2.5	2.75	3.25	3.5	3.75	4	
Overcoming Shyness (11 + 25 + 35 + 49) / 4		No norms available. I suggest "2.0" may imply a "slight need," "3.0" a "moderate need," and "4.0" a great need.									
Overcoming Social Anxiety (Experimental Scale) (10 + 16 + 28 + 38 + 59) / 5		No norms available. I suggest "2.0" may imply a "slight need," "3.0" a "moderate need," and "4.0" a great need.									
Relating Assertively (6 + 19 + 29 + 37 + 54) / 5	2.45 (.75)	1.4	1.8	2	2.2	2.4	2.5	2.8	3	3.4	4
Managing Anger (13 + 22 + 33 + 43) / 4	2.68 (.85)		1	1.5	1.75	2	2.25	2.75	3	3.5	4
Managing Anxiety (3 + 41) / 2	1.80 (.73)			1		1.5		2	2.5	3	4
Managing Depression (15 + 45) / 2	1.74 (.73)			1		1.5		2	2.5	3	4
Coping with Symptoms of Skeletal Muscle Tension (7 + 20 + 32 + 48) / 4	1.89 (.71)	1	1.25	1.38	1.5	1.75	2	2.25	2.5	2.75	4
Coping with Symptoms of Autonomic Arousal (4 + 14 + 23 + 34 + 44 + 50 +58) / 7	1.56 (.46)	1	1.14		1.29	1.42	1.57	1.71	2	2.14	4
Coping with Pain (5 + 18 + 26 + 39) / 4	2.08 (.83)	1	1.25	1.5	1.75	2	2.25	2.5	2.75	3.25	4

NORM SAMPLE: 273 males; 924 females; age = 28.99 yrs (sd = 8.10). Participants recruited from undergraduate classes) psychology and other; at twelve Chicago and Illinois junior and four-year colleges. Chronbach alphas (combined sample): Relaxation ≥ .80, Problems ≥ .80, Time = .86, Worry = .82, Shyness = .82, Social anxiety = .85, Social anxiety = Not Available, Assertive = .79, Anger = .87, Anxiety = .55, Depression = .81. Skeletal = .74, Autonomic Arousal = .70. Pain = .74.

FIGURE 1.1 SSMMI scoring key and norms for males.

SCALES (Scoring Key)

INSTRUCTIONS: Add items in parentheses. Then divide the sum by the number to the right of the "/" mark. Thus, to obtain one's score for the "Managing Anxiety" scale, first add the responses to items 3 and 41. Then divide this by 2. Finally, find the appropriate match in the "ESTIMATED PERCENTILES" table to the right.

ESTIMATED PERCENTILES

For each scale, find percentile score below that most closely matches SCOREBOX score. If there is no exact match, select closest lower percentile score. Percentile means "Score is higher than X% of sample."

SCALES (Scoring Key)	M (sd)	SCOREBOX	10	20	30	40	50	60	70	80	90	100
SMITH STRESS MANAGEMENT MOTIVATIONS INVENTORY												
Relaxation (8 + 31 + 51) / 3												
Solving Problems and Negotiating (1 + 9 + 21 + 27 + 36 + 42 + 47 + 53 + 56) / 9	2.34 (.75)		1.33	1.66	1.89	2.11	2.33	2.53	2.78	3	3.36	4
Managing Time and Dealing with Procrastination (17 + 30 + 46 + 55 + 57) / 5	2.63 (.91)		1.2	1.8	2	2.4	2.6	3	3.2	3.6	4	
Managing Worry (2 + 12 + 24 + 40 + 52) / 5	2.55 (.92)		1.4	1.8	2	2.4	2.6	2.8	3	3.4	3.6	4
Overcoming Shyness (11 + 25 + 35 + 49) / 4	2.40 (.92)		1	1.5	1.75	2	2.5	2.75	3	3.25	3.75	4
Overcoming Social Anxiety (Experimental Scale) (10 + 16 + 28 + 38 + 59) / 5			No norms available. I suggest "2.0" may imply a "slight need," "3.0" a "moderate need," and "4.0" a great need.									
Relating Assertively (6 + 19 + 29 + 37 + 54) / 5	2.57 (.83)		1.4	1.8	2.02	2.4	2.6	2.8	3	3.4	3.6	4
Managing Anger (13 + 22 + 33 + 43) / 4	2.29 (.91)		1	1.25	1.75	2	2.25	2.5	2.75	3.25	3.75	4
Managing Anxiety (3 + 41) / 2	1.85 (.77)			1			1.5		2	2.5	3	4
Managing Depression (15 + 45) / 2	1.83 (.88)				1		1.5		2	2.5	3.5	4
Coping with Symptoms of Skeletal Muscle Tension (7 + 20 + 32 + 48) / 4	2.17 (.82)		1.25	1.5		1.75	2	2.25	2.5	3	3.5	4
Coping with Symptoms of Autonomic Arousal (4 + 14 + 23 + 34 + 44 + 50 +58) / 7	1.59 (.53)		1	1.14		1.29	1.42	1.57	1.86	2	2.29	4
Coping with Pain (5 + 18 + 26 + 39) / 4	2.09 (.83)		1	1.25	1.5	1.75	2	2.25	2.25	2.75	3.25	4

FIGURE 1.2   SSMMI scoring key and norms for females.

Managing Worry

Problems with excessive, uncontrollable, and intrusive worry are typically surface indicators of deeper problems with distorted thinking. Specific irrational beliefs can be assessed by the Smith Irrational Beliefs Inventory (SIBI), presented in chapter 6 (key chapters: 6, 4; supplementary chapter: 14).

Overcoming Shyness

Shyness is often a problem for young adults, although similar issues can be present at any age. Immediate specific concerns include meeting others and developing and maintaining relationships (key chapters: 10, 4, 6, 5, 8, 7; supplementary chapter: 9).

Overcoming Social Anxiety

Social anxiety refers to self-conscious tension and discomfort one feels in public situations in which one is observed while performing an activity (public speaking, music performance, sports, eating, even making mistakes). This scale is experimental. Scoring criteria are suggestive, not norm-based (key chapters: 10, 4, 6, 8, 7; supplementary chapter: 9).

Relating Assertively

To be assertive is to honestly and appropriately express one's wants, thoughts, and feelings while respecting others. Specifically, our research shows that those who express a desire to be more assertive typically want to develop skills at effectively expressing feelings and wants, saying no to requests of others, and responding to behavior that is objectionable or hostile (key chapter: 8; supplementary chapters: 6, 7, 9, 11).

Managing Anger

Individuals with problems managing anger express a desire to control and reduce destructive anger and to respond assertively and productively when anger is provoked (key chapters: 11, 6, 4; supplementary chapters: 5, 8, 9).

Managing Anxiety

Individuals who generally desire to reduce excessive feelings of fear and anxiety often have more specific concerns assessed by other SSMMI scales (key chapters: 4, 6, 7; supplementary chapter: 5).

Managing Depression

As with anxiety, reports of distressing depression are often accompanied by more specific needs reflected in other scales (key chapter: 6; supplementary chapters: 4, 5, 14).

Coping with Symptoms of Skeletal Muscle Tension

The skeletal muscles include those muscles over which one has direct "voluntary" control, including muscles used for walking, moving, lifting, etc. Research strongly suggests that progressive muscle relaxation, yoga stretching, and possibly autogenic training techniques targeted to specific areas of muscle tension can be particularly effective (key chapter: 4).

Coping with Symptoms of Autonomic Arousal

Autonomic arousal is manifest in symptoms involving organs and body systems over which one ordinarily does not have direct control (except after professional biofeedback or relaxation training). Symptoms include rapidly beating heart, shallowness of breath, and excessive perspiration. Often these symptoms are direct manifestations of the stress arousal "fight-or-flight" response as discussed in chapter 2 (key chapter: 4; supplementary chapters: 5, 6, 7).

Coping with Pain

This is not a text on pain management. However, a brief pain symptom scale is included to identify clients who may benefit from pain management treatment provided by a specialist. Such strategies include, but are not limited to, all of the approaches covered in this text. (Key chapters: 4, 6, 7; supplementary chapter: 5; additional professional assistance is recommended).

Finally, it is my profound bias that virtually all stress-related problems can benefit from some form of professional relaxation training. For this reason, all clients and students should read chapter 4, and all psychologists, counselors, social workers, psychiatrists, rehabilitation specialists, and health professionals should read : *ABC Relaxation Theory: An Evidence-Based Approach, ABC Relaxation Training, A Practical Guide for Health Professionals,* and *Advances in ABC Relaxation: Applications and Inventories* (Springer Publishing Company, New York).

2

Stress Concepts

Stress is wear and tear brought on by perceived threats and coping deficiencies. The first step in stress management is realizing what stress is, that one is indeed under stress, and what the contributing factors might be.

Most people have a fragmented understanding of stress in their lives. For example, examine the following situations:

CORPORATE SECRETARY: "Stress for me is feeling tense in my shoulders. "

BUS DRIVER: "Stress is my nutty boss! He doesn't give me any respect."

COLLEGE STUDENT: "I'm always worrying. I guess I'm just a nervous type of person."

BANKING VICE PRESIDENT: "I feel under stress whenever I feel stuck and helpless."

Each of these accounts focuses on some part of our definition of stress, whether it be physical or emotional wear and tear (tension in shoulders, worry, nervousness), perceived threats (nutty bosses, not receiving respect), or not having the skills or resources to manage problems (feeling stuck and helpless). However, each person has left out important information. Our corporate secretary says, "Stress for me is feeling tense in my shoulders." Her understanding does not include what is causing the tension and what she has tried to do about it. Our bus driver troubled by his "nutty boss" is telling us only part of the story. Has he contributed to the problem in any way? Our college student says, "I'm always worrying." Worrying about what? How serious is this problem? Is it getting in the way of studying or socializing after school? And our banking vice president describes her problem as feeling "stuck and helpless." Why? How has she tried and failed to deal with her stress problems? Fragmented understandings of stress miss the entire story.

THE SIX STRESS VARIABLES

Stress is not just one thing—a symptom, event, or problem. Stress is a complex combination of six types of variables:

1. Stressors (stress events or situations),
2. Distorted stressful appraisals,
3. Physiological arousal,
4. Medical and emotional distress,
5. Reduced psychological functioning, and
6. Coping deficiencies

A complete picture of our bus driver (with the "nutty boss") might read like this (each type of variable is highlighted in parentheses):

> Stress is my nutty boss. He doesn't give me any respect. Yesterday I helped an elderly woman off the bus, and this slowed down my schedule by 30 minutes *(stressor)*. When I finished late, my boss criticized me without first asking what happened. I really felt bad. I was sure I was going to lose my job and that everyone would think that I was wasting time *(distorted stressful appraisal)*. I started getting a stomachache *(physiological arousal)* and my ulcer started acting up *(medical distress)*. I felt really blue and depressed *(emotional distress)*. The next day at work, my mind just wasn't on the job and I drove slower than usual *(reduced psychological functioning)*. I took Friday off and spent time at the bar, but that didn't help *(coping deficiency)*.

We now consider each type of stress variable.

1. Stressors (Stress Events or Situations)

Thomas Holmes and Richard Rahe (1967) were among the first researchers to examine stress. They proposed that stressors can be defined as life situations and events that call for change and readjustment and as a result can contribute to illness. The Holmes and Rahe *Social Readjustment Rating Scale* is an early stress test consisting of 43 life events. Here are some examples:

Death of spouse 100
Divorce 73
Jail term 63
Personal injury or illness 53

Marriage. 50
Retirement 45
Gain of new family member. 39
Son or daughter leaving home. 29
Change in residence 20
Christmas. 12
Minor violations of the law. 11

The weight to the right of each stressor indicates the average amount of change and readjustment the event presumably evokes, suggested by Holmes and Rahe. Early stress researchers postulated that change and readjustment in and of itself is enough to create wear and tear and contribute to stress-related illness, much as excessive use can stress a household appliance.

To take the Social Readjustment Rating Scale, one checks the stressors experienced over the last six months and adds up the change and readjustment scores for the events. The total score is an indicator of how much stress has been experienced.

The Social Readjustment Rating Scale has been subjected to considerable criticism. Stress researchers have found that other factors must be considered if we are to understand how much stress a person is under. First, even minor events, or *hassles,* can be stressful (Lazarus & Folkman, 1984). Such everyday problems as "trouble relaxing," "misplacing or losing things," "not enough time for family," and "too many things to do" can add up. *Central hassles,* those that reflect important ongoing themes or problems in a person's life, appear to be more stressful (Gruen, Folkman, & Lazarus, 1988). In addition we must consider a person's stressful appraisals, coping deficiencies, physiological arousal, and distress, variables we will discuss later in this chapter.

However, knowing what life events people have encountered can help us understand how much stress they might be under. Researchers have identified five life event and hassle attributes or "danger signs" that can warn of possible problems (Smith, 1993a; Thoits, 1983). The most important are:

Unpredictability. Was the event or hassle unexpected?
Uncontrollability. Was it something over which one had little control?

If an event is unpredictable or uncontrollable, it can be rendered more severe by:

Undesirability. Was the life event or hassle something one did not want?

Magnitude. Was the event or hassle important or large?

Clustering. Did several events or hassles happen at about the same time?

Finally, all of these variables can be aggravated by stressor proximity and duration. Long-lasting and chronic stressors which directly impact an individual are most severe.

2. Distorted Stressful Appraisals

Popular culture often tells us that "stress is all in the mind" or "how you think creates stress." Such notions are oversimplified; a complete understanding of stress must also consider life events and hassles, arousal, coping deficiencies, functioning, and distress. However, popular wisdom carries a grain of truth.

Richard Lazarus (1984) has identified two types of stress-related thinking. *Primary appraisal* concerns the stakes a person has in a stressful encounter. How are a person's wants or needs endangered? Does he or she feel harmed, or merely threatened by a potential harm? Perhaps one views stress as a challenge, with some potential for good. *Secondary appraisal* concerns the options and prospects for coping. One asks, "What, if anything, can be done about my stressful situation?" When a person thinks a situation is threatening, and thinks he or she can't deal with it, he or she is displaying stressful primary and secondary appraisal.

Not all forms of primary and secondary appraisal are equally stressful. Compare the following problems:

PERSON 1: "I wanted that raise this year; I thought about asking my boss for one, but I knew it wouldn't make any difference."

PERSON 2: "I wanted that raise this year; I thought about asking my boss for one, but I knew it wouldn't make any difference. This is a catastrophe for me, the end of the world. I can't seem to get anything I want. I should just quit trying."

Both problem descriptions reflect the same primary and secondary appraisals. The primary appraisal is "I wanted a raise and didn't get it." The secondary appraisal is "I thought I couldn't do anything about it." However, our second example shows considerably more stress. Why?

Albert Ellis (1962, 1985) and Aaron Beck (1976) have noted that appraisals are most likely to be stressful when they are *irrational* and *maladaptive,* that is, when they run counter to the facts or reason, and simply get in the way of good coping. In the examples we just considered, the thought "This is a catastrophe for me, the end of the world" is most likely irrational. Few events merit the label "catastrophe." It is more sensible to recognize the failure to get a raise as an irritation or frustration (perhaps a "hassle"), but not comparable to the catastrophes of war and famine. And the appraisal, "I can't seem to get anything I want. I should just quit trying" is maladaptive, or not particularly helpful. As long as our person keeps thinking about giving up, he probably will not succeed.

3. Physiological Arousal

It takes energy to deal with the problems of living. A football player running to the goalpost, a letter carrier fighting off a barking dog, and a camper lifting a fallen tree off the leg of a partner each display the human capacity for extraordinary feats of effort. Each of us has an automatic physiological response that awakens and energizes us for emergency action. Physiologist Walter Cannon (1929) called this the *fight-or-flight response.* Our ancestors in the wild hardly had time to figure out how to ready their bodies to fight off an attacking gorilla. Fortunately, our brains do this automatically. When triggered by the hypothalamus, a cluster of nerves deep in the brain, a constellation of changes take place:

- Sugars, fats, and proteins are released for energy.
- Increased breathing rate brings in oxygen to "burn" fuel.
- Heartbeat and blood pressure increase; blood vessels expand, more blood is pumped to hard-working muscles.
- As workload increases, heat is carried away through breathing and perspiration.
- Nonessential functions are reduced, including gastrointestinal activity and blood flow to the skin.
- To prepare for possible injury and bleeding, surface blood vessels constrict, and clotting substances are released into the blood (for scarring).
- The immune system becomes more active to prepare for infection, or becomes less active to reduce the infection and conserve energy.
- The brain's painkillers, *endorphins,* minimize the distracting discomfort of injury.
- Muscle tone increases, eye pupils enlarge (letting more light in), palms and feet become moist (increasing grip and traction)—all enhancing one's ability to engage in vigorous physical activity.

People often experience a variety of symptoms that can indicate stress arousal, including:

- Fast, hard, irregular heartbeat
- Hurried, shallow, or uneven breathing

- Tight, tense, or clenched up (furrowed brow, making fist, clenching jaws, etc.) muscles
- Restlessness and fidgetiness
- Tension and self-consciousness when saying or doing something
- Perspiring or feeling too warm
- Feeling the need to go the rest room
- Feeling uncoordinated
- Dry mouth
- Fatigue
- Headache
- Feeling unfit or heavy
- Backache
- Shoulders, neck, or back feels tense
- Worsened skin condition (blemishes, oiliness)
- Watering or tearing eyes
- Nervous stomach
- Loss of appetite

People may think of stress as always negative. The fight-or-flight response can be very useful, however, even life saving. It provides quick energy for the football player catching a pass, the secretary who must prepare for an immediate emergency, and the jogger running from a dog in the park.

However, the fight-or-flight response can also be triggered by non-emergencies such as alarm clocks, worries, interpersonal conflict, and excessive work. In such cases, stress energy increases and is not discharged through vigorous emergency action. Over days and weeks, stress arousal continues to rise, eventually contributing to distress on body organs and illness.

It should be emphasized that one can be unaware of stress arousal through habituation. The brain can tune out constant, unchanging stimuli, whether it be the background drone of air conditioners, traffic noise, or stress. Indeed, one goal of stress management is to sensitize people to symptoms they may be missing so they can tell when they are under stress and when stress management is working.

4. Medical and Emotional Distress

Hans Seyle (1956) has coined two useful terms that help us understand stress: eustress and distress. Put simply, eustress is positive and constructive; distress is negative and destructive. Distress provides people with important information about the severity of stress in their lives. We consider two types: medical and emotional.

Medical Distress

We have seen that stress arousal, the high-energy fight-or-flight response, prepares us for emergency action. In today's world, this response is often activated repeatedly without relief. Chronic stress arousal can contribute to medical problems in at least two ways. High levels of chronic arousal are not healthy, and just as driving an automobile all day at high speed can lead to early mechanical problems (in addition to possible arrest), stress can contribute to strain and dysfunction in just about any bodily system, contributing to gastrointestinal problems, back pain, and so on. Also, chronic arousal suppresses the ability of the immune system to protect against and recover from illness. In sum, stress can increase vulnerability to, aggravate, and prolong a wide range of illnesses, including:

- AIDS/HIV infection
- allergies
- arthritis
- atherosclerosis
- bruxism
- cancer
- chronic lung disease
- cirrhosis of the liver
- diabetes
- headache
- heart palpitations
- hypertension
- influenza
- irritable colon
- kidney impairment
- pneumonia
- skin disorders
- sleep disorders
- stroke
- ulcers

The mechanisms by which stress contributes to illness are beyond the scope of this book. If you are interested in learning more, consult my book, *Understanding Stress and Coping* (Smith, 1993b) or a good recent text in health psychology.

Emotional Distress

Among the best indicators of psychological distress are negative emotions (Lazarus & Folkman, 1984), generally anxiety, depression, and anger (Plutchik, 1994). *Anxiety* can include feelings of fearfulness, threat, panic, dread, and tension. Feelings of *depression* include sadness, shame, guilt, hopelessness, dejection, despondency, discouragement, and sorrow. *Anger* covers a broad range of feelings, including hostility, resentment, irritability, and cynicism.

People often experience emotion in complex ways. Various emotions can be combined, for example, feeling angry and depressed at the same time. Some emotions are the "tip of an iceberg" of a wide range of other, hidden feelings. For example, a person may at first describe feeling depressed. After sharing and exploring this feeling, one may uncover a variety of hidden feelings, perhaps guilt and fear.

5. Reduced Psychological Functioning

Excessive stress can interfere with our ability to do our best, at work and play and when relating to others. Such problems can include minor lapses in memory, inflexibility, inability to think creatively, decreased interpersonal sensitivity, accidents, and errors in performance. Severe deficits in psychological functioning include inability to continue work or school, form or keep satisfying relationships, or take care of oneself or others.

Stress can interfere with psychological functioning in a variety of ways. Different tasks require different levels of arousal; high arousal may actually help one complete a task requiring brute strength and endurance, but interfere with tasks requiring thought and coordination. Too much stress can narrow one's attention, leading one to think rigidly and miss subtle details. Stress may lead one to focus less on present tasks and become preoccupied with distraction and negative emotion. Finally, stress can interfere with complex interpersonal and problem-solving skills.

6. Coping Deficiencies

It is easy to confuse coping, stress management, appraisal, and functioning. First, we consider stress management to be a limited form of coping, a set of coping skills as taught in a stress management classroom or clinic; coping refers to the application of such skills (with or without prior training) in life at large.

To continue, cognitive appraisals include two types of thoughts, those concerning the stakes one has in a stressful encounter and the options and prospects for coping. In contrast, coping refers to deeds, attempts to change oneself or a stressful situation. And functioning refers to how well we complete our deeds. We can see these distinctions in the following example:

> This year I did not receive the promotion I expected. I really counted on the extra income and am not sure how I can make ends meet (appraisal). To make things worse, I am concerned that my wife will

think I'm goofing off at work (appraisal). I decided to do something about it and talk to my boss. I wrote out a list of my concerns and made an appointment to see him (coping). I don't know what went wrong. I guess I got cold feet and called in "sick" the day of the appointment, even though I was fine (functioning).

The distinction between maladaptive coping and low functioning can be a bit arbitrary. In the example we just considered, "calling in sick" was presented as an example of poor functioning, in that it reflected a deficiency in one's ability to carry out a planned course of action. This behavior could also be seen as a maladaptive form of coping. For example, perhaps the prospect of confronting the boss creates anxiety, and our worker decided to cope with this anxiety by simply not showing up for work. Generally, a behavior reflects maladaptive coping if you can identify how it attempts to reduce some threat or minimize some harm; it reflects low functioning if it simply reflects a performance deficit with no apparent gain.

Lazarus (Lazarus & Folkman, 1984) has defined two types of coping: *problem focused coping*, or trying to actually alter a stressful situation, and *emotion-focused coping*, or reducing the upset or discomfort associated with a stressful situation without actively trying to change the situation itself. Stress researchers have expanded this distinction with a variety of lists of coping strategies people use. These strategies can be sorted into four categories, depending on whether we (1) actively attempt to change a stressful situation, (2) alter how we realistically appraise or think of the situation, (3) release pent-up emotions and tension or simply relax, or (4) distort and deny the existence or severity of a problem or withdraw from the problem.

STRESS EQUATIONS, STRESS VARIABLES, AND STRESS STORIES

A complete understanding of personal stress incorporates the six stress variables we have discussed. Even such a comprehensive approach can be oversimplified. For example, one might be tempted to insert stress variables into an equation suggesting limited one-way cause–effect relationships. For example, one might think that stressors → distorted appraisals → arousal → distress → reduced functioning → coping deficiencies. However, like any good story, stress stories are often complex. Each part can influence other parts in unexpected ways. Criticism at work (a stressor) might trigger stomach distress (medical distress), which provokes worries about health (appraisal), which distracts one from working more efficiently and considering coping options (coping deficiencies), leading to further criticism from the boss.

No one single stress equation fits everyone. Different people experience stress differently, and differently from day to day, hour to hour. The stress management techniques and strategies offered in this book are equally diverse; no one chapter works for everyone, and different combinations of chapters, often in different orders, work for different people. However, taken together the ideas and skills we will explore offer opportunities for more effective coping in life at large.

EXERCISES

1. Identify a stressor in your life. Which of the event and hassle attributes made it worse (undesirability, unpredictability, uncontrollability, magnitude, clustering)? Why?
2. What arousal signs do you notice when under stress?
3. Can you think of any recent illness you have had that might have been stress-related? Why?
4. Do you know of anyone who has had what you suspect was a stress-related illness? Explain.
5. Think of a time when excess stress impaired your ability to do your best at home or school. How did stress interfere (refer to Part 5, "Reduced Psychological Functioning")?
6. Can you recall a situation in which you noted stress impairing the performance of someone else? Explain.
7. Think of a recent situation in which you, or someone you know, displayed emotion-focused coping or problem-focused coping. Describe the situation. Explain the costs and benefits of the coping displayed.

In the following stress stories, see what types of information are presented. What important facts are missing? Why might it be important to know something about the missing information?

Person 1: "I've just started college and have run into some trouble. I can't seem to get my grades up. I've got to pass my courses, otherwise my job won't reimburse me for tuition. And if I don't get my degree, I won't get that promotion. This really upsets me. I get so anxious that I sit for hours just thinking about what might go wrong if I don't straighten out. I don't know what's going wrong. I attend every class. I spend about an hour each night reading my books. I got good grades in high school. It's tougher now studying. I have two roommates, and both like to stay up late partying. They don't realize that I have to go to school and work at the same time. I wish they were more considerate; people should just know when their lack of sensitivity is hurting others. Sometimes I don't get enough sleep and am tired the next day. But I pull through at work. I guess I don't really need that much sleep."

Person 2: "My boyfriend and I just can't communicate. He yells at me and calls me stupid, and that makes me wonder if he loves me. Then, the same night he kisses and makes up. Like this week when I dented the car. Little problem. I would pay for it. But I knew it would be a big thing. He just blew up and called me a 'stupid blond.' I started thinking, 'Oh my God, he wants to break up. What will I do? I can't live without him.' I got so jittery I started stammering. I finally cooled off by watching my favorite soap opera. Jill, my friend, called and asked if anything was wrong. I said, 'Oh, I'm fine.' I didn't want her to think I'm crazy and not talk to me any more. Then, after dinner, my boyfriend hugged me and said how much he loved me. The same old cycle. And I am left feeling like I'm on a roller coaster. I feel like such a child. I guess I think people should just know when they're hurting the feelings of others."

3

Crises, Catastrophes, and Acute Stress Disorder

We end our introduction to stress basics and begin our exploration of stress management with stress in its purest form. Traumatic events are severe and extraordinary stressors outside the realm of normal human experience, events that unfortunately have emerged as particularly salient in our age. Examples range from human acts of terror and environmental disaster to rape, robbery, and illness (see Table 3.1). Reactions to such events often reveal and illuminate, in the bright light of crisis, processes that underlie all stress and coping. In this chapter we conclude our overview of stress basics and introduce stress management with a discussion of acute stress disorder (American Psychiatric Association, *Diagnostic and Statistical Manual of Mental Disorders,* Fourth Edition, Text Revision; DSM-IV-TR, 2000).

ACUTE STRESS DISORDER

A person with acute stress disorder has experienced a traumatic event with feelings of intense fear, helplessness, or horror. In addition, one displays four clusters of symptoms that represent a special pattern of the fundamental stress variables considered in chapter 2: (1) dissociation, (2) reexperiencing the trauma, (3) avoidance, and (4) hyperarousal. The following summary represents an integration of various sources, including the American Psychiatric Association (2000), Friedman (2000), and Schiraldi (2000).

1. *Dissociation* is the most prominent symptom and reflects a significant and abnormal alteration of how one perceives oneself and the environment. DSM-IV specifies five categories of dissociation, three of which must be present before a diagnosis of acute stress disorder can be applied:

TABLE 3.1   Examples of Stressors Outside the Realm of Normal Human Experience

Deliberate Human Activities
- Terrorist attack
- Breakdown of social infrastructure (mail delivery system; health system; air transportation; communication network; energy, food, and water resources)
- Bombing
- Riot
- Military combat
- Sexual assault
- Sexual abuse
- Physical attack
- Serious physical abuse
- Robbery
- Mugging
- Kidnapping
- Being taken hostage
- Torture
- Involuntary incarceration
- Suicide/death

Unintentional Human Activities (accidents, technological disaster)
- Serious automobile accident
- Serious industrial accident
- Serious sports/recreational accident
- Breakdown of social infrastructure (mail delivery system, health system, air transportation, communication network)—if not due to terrorist attack
- Nuclear power plant disaster
- Surgical damage to body
- Fires and explosions
- Plane crash
- Train wreck
- Boating accident/shipwreck
- Building/ major structure collapse

Acts of Nature/Natural Disaster
- Earthquake
- Flood
- Global warming
- Epidemic/plague (not human origin)
- Meteor/comet catastrophe
- Hurricane/tornado
- Heat wave
- Severe snow/rain
- Avalanche/mudslide
- Brushfire
- Famine
- Sinkholes

TABLE 3.1 *(Continued)*

- Animal (wild dog/cat, bear) attack
- Severe illness or medical incident (heart attack)
- Death of loved one

One need not be a direct victim to experience the impact of crises and catastrophes; traumatic events can be witnessed or learned about through word of mouth, television, radio, the Internet, or the print media.

Note: Incorporates ideas suggested by Bryant & Harvey (2000), Caplan (1964), Friedman (2000), Horowitz (1982), Schiraldi (2000), and Slaikeu (1990), as well as the American Psychiatric Association, *Diagnostic and Statistical Manual of Mental Disorders*, 4th ed. text revision (2000).

A. *Psychic numbing.* Immediately after a trauma, one might have feelings of numbing, detachment, lack of involvement in life, or absence of emotional responsiveness. One might have difficulty loving, crying, laughing, caring, or even feeling anger. Previously enjoyed activities are no longer a source of fun and pleasure. Numbing is a psychological defense mechanism in which one tunes out all feelings in order to tune out painful feelings related to a trauma.

B. *Reduced awareness of surroundings.* One might experience being "in a daze," "spaced out," or "in one's own private world" and simply not notice or respond to other people, events, or other environmental stimuli. As with numbing, reduced awareness is a wholesale strategy that enables one to tune out traumatic pain.

C. *Derealization.* One may feel detached from one's familiar world. Things and people may seem unfamiliar, strange, unreal, dreamlike, or mechanical. There might be a sense of seeing things as if they were not really happening. One might feel like a stranger or an outsider, even in familiar places. Sometimes derealization is associated with a distorted sense of time in which events seem speeded up or slowed down. Derealization may be both an attempt to distance oneself from a trauma and a secondary effect of numbing and reduced awareness.

D. *Depersonalization.* One may experience distortions in how one sees one's body or self. Examples include "out of body experiences" in which one has the experience of being separated from one's body, perhaps looking down from above or across the room, or watching a movie of oneself. The body might be sensed as split into parts, or one part of the body might feel numb, warm, or cold. Depersonalization, like derealization, serves to distance oneself from trauma.

E. *Dissociative amnesia.* One might be unable to remember an important aspect of a traumatic event.

2. *Reexperiencing the trauma* can occur in a variety of ways. One might have recurrent mental images or fantasies, thoughts, dreams, nightmares, or illusions. In flashback episodes a trauma may be reexperienced or "replayed" mentally. Flashbacks are predominantly visual, and can be so vivid that one actually thinks he or she is reliving an event; however, they are often quickly forgotten. They can be triggered by insomnia, fatigue, stress arousal, drugs, or deep relaxation. Also, stimuli that remind one of the traumatic event may evoke psychological or physical distress. Such reminders might be seen as unwelcome and painful intrusions, outside of one's control, and consequently evoke fear, vulnerability, rage, or other feelings of distress.

3. One might display marked *avoidance of stimuli* that stir recollections of the trauma. This can include avoiding thoughts, feelings, conversations, activities, places, and people. Although avoidance and dissociation are often coping strategies for reducing experience of a trauma, avoidance is usually under one's conscious control whereas dissociation is unconscious and automatic.

4. *Hyperarousal* is an exaggerated and prolonged manifestation of the stress arousal "fight-or-flight response" we considered in chapter 2. It includes such symptoms as difficulty sleeping (because one is so tense), irritability (including emotional outbursts, arguing, flying off the handle, intense criticizing or impatience), poor concentration and memory, exaggerated startle response (overreact, jump, tense up, or flinch when startled), and physical restlessness (fidgeting, pacing, etc.). Hyperarousal may be manifest as hypervigilance, or a heightened sensitivity and feelings of "being on guard." Schiraldi (2000) notes other important signs of hypervigilance:

- feeling vulnerable, fearful of lots of things, unable to feel calm in safe places
- fear or repetition
- anticipating disaster; needing to sit in the corner of a room with back to the wall—looking for exits, places to hide . . .
- rapid scanning, looking over one's shoulder
- keeping a weapon or several weapons
- being overprotective or overcontrolling of loved ones (p. 9)

Other hyperarousal symptoms include all of those noted in chapter 2.

An acute stress reaction is a serious response to trauma. It must last for a minimum of two days and no more than a month. If symptoms last more than a month, then another, more serious diagnosis should be considered, perhaps post traumatic stress disorder (PTSD). In addition, one displays significant distress or impairment in social, occupation, or other important areas of functioning. One's coping ability is impaired, and one might find it difficult to complete tasks necessary for survival (going to work, protecting oneself and family, seeking help).

ACUTE STRESS DISORDER AND THE SIX STRESS VARIABLES

Acute stress disorder provides a vivid illustration of the six basic stress variables we considered in chapter 2:

1. Stressors (stress events or situations)
2. Distorted stressful appraisals
3. Physiological arousal,
4. Medical and emotional distress,
5. Reduced psychological functioning, and
6. Coping deficiencies

A traumatic event can display all those characteristics that define stressor severity, including uncontrollability, unpredictability, undesirability, magnitude, and clustering. Symptoms of arousal (hyperarousal) and distress are central to this disorder. We see significantly impaired functioning. However, what is particularly interesting is the specific manifestation of appraisal and coping.

ACUTE STRESS DISORDER, APPRAISAL, AND COPING

There are many ways of conceptualizing the symptoms that define acute stress disorder. We consider a perspective that has had considerable impact on the field.

A traumatic event can be seen as a crisis, "a temporary state of upset and disorganization, characterized chiefly by an individual's inability to cope with a particular situation using customary methods of problem solving, and by the potential for a radically positive or negative outcome." (Slaiken, 1990, p. 15). To elaborate, one may progress through various stages of coping (Caplan, 1964) that begin with applying existing habitual coping strategies. If these fail, tension increases and other, less familiar coping strategies may be risked, or personal goals redefined or abandoned. When these strategies fail, tension increases, and one experiences emotional disorganization, disequilibrium, and suggestibility. One may feel increasingly helpless, vulnerable, and filled with grief. Functioning may deteriorate. At this state one may be especially suggestible and open to influences (both constructive and destructive) of others.

Part of the task of dealing with a crisis is similar to the task of stress management—relaxing, solving problems, thinking realistically, and so on. Particularly important is the goal of *working through* intense emotional upset. Horowitz (1982) has presented a useful model of this process.

One's first reaction to a crisis is intense emotional shock or outcry, such as fainting, weeping, or panic. Physical and mental arousal may increase, potentially disrupting the working through process. The real "work" of working through consists of a dosing process in which one alternates between phases of intrusion and denial, or as I prefer, approach and withdrawal. During periods of approach, one moves intellectually and emotionally closer to the crisis event and reexperiences the event. In the withdrawal phase, one moves away from the crisis event and is less likely to experience associated thoughts or feelings. This can be reflected in dissociation or avoidance.

What is important to recognize is that alternating phases of approach and withdrawal, or intrusion and denial, are part of a working through process in which one is dosed with manageable pieces of a crisis. Put differently, a terrorist attack, disaster, loss of a loved one, or illness may have far too many emotional ramifications to be dealt with at once. For example, after losing one's house to a fire one might have to deal with the emotions of fear, rage, and depression as well as the tasks of finding new housing, dealing with the feelings of family and loved ones, and so on. Through dosing, one approaches the crisis, deals with one part of the problem at a time, and withdraws to recover and regroup. When ready, one may spontaneously experience additional approach and intrusion.

The eventual goal of such working through is to emotionally and intellectually accept the facts of a crisis, and learn to go on living and coping. Often specific intense emotional issues must be uncovered, experienced, and dealt with, including

1. fear of repetition,
2. shame over being helpless,
3. rage at perceived "sources" of the crisis,
4. intense general anger,
5. guilt over being a survivor ("why me? I am not deserving."), and
6. simple sadness over serious loss.

In order for such feelings to be processed for potential distorted thinking, accepted, and put aside, they must be first experienced (approach or intrusion). One can then go on living, hopefully with enhanced coping skills.

WORKING WITH CLIENTS EXPERIENCING ACUTE STRESS DISORDER: STRESS MANAGEMENT GOALS

Stress management treatments directed to clients with acute stress disorder have a number of objectives. Short-term goals include:

1. To resolve any problems that immediately threaten the client's life, health, or well-being. For example, does the client have food and housing for the night? Is he or she out of harm's way? Is there a risk for suicide (this requires professional assessment beyond the scope of this book; if a client discusses or threatens suicide, professional assistance must be immediately sought).

2. To marshal any resources immediately necessary for maintaining life, health, or well-being. Does the client have reliable food and safe housing?

Both of these objectives can require direct application of systematic problem solving (chapter 5) and assertiveness (chapter 8). Secondarily, the client may require assistance in overcoming procrastination (chapter 13), or dealing with shyness that may interfere with gaining assistance (chapter 10).

Longer term goals involve (Bryand & Harvey, 2000; Caplan, 1964; Horowitz, 1982; Slaikeu, 1990):

1. To accept the event,
2. To learn to put the event aside so it is no longer a pressing concern, and
3. To go on coping and live and full and satisfying life. This involves viewing the world as reasonably safe, predictable, and controllable and trusting one's coping resources.

To these ends, the full array of stress management skills in this text can be useful.

PSYCHOLOGICAL DEBRIEFING AND STRESS MANAGEMENT

Once short-term goals are met, formal stress management of acute stress disorder can begin. The clinician must first establish a treatment environment and relationship characterized by trust and safety. These cannot be forced upon a client, but must be earned through respect and empathic listening (chapter 9). Friedman (2000) noted that a variety of treatments are available designed for immediate application to a traumatized individual (notably critical incident stress debriefing, Mitchell, 1983). Generally summarized as psychological debriefing, they are ideally conducted in a place and at a time close to the actual trauma. Psychological debriefing is typically conducted in groups of 10 to 20 and involves six basic stages, which I have adapted to incorporate concepts and techniques in this book:

1. *Introduction.* The group leader introduces him or herself and establishes the rules of confidentiality, mutual respect, and openness.

2. *Expectations and facts.* The group discusses what they witnessed, and what they expected would happen. Different members provide different perspectives. The focus is on facts, "who, what, where, and when" (chapter 5).

3. *Thoughts and impressions.* Members then describe their thoughts and sensory impressions of the event.

4. *Emotional reactions.* Painful and often unexpressed emotional reactions are then shared. Empathy (chapter 9) can be a powerful tool to facilitate this process. Enabling one to fully work through painful emotions without interruption is a key treatment objective (exposure, chapter 7).

5. *Education.* The venting of emotions enables participants to learn that others have had other similar reactions, and that such reactions are normal. At this point, the group leader may introduce relevant facts from chapter 2 and this chapter.

6. *Future planning/referral.* The group leader reviews future emotional and coping problems participants may experience (chapter 2, this chapter) and briefly reviews stress management strategies that may be appropriate (relaxation, chapter 4; problem-solving, chapter 5; cognitive change, chapter 6; review and rehearsal, chapter 7; assertiveness, chapter 8; empathic listening, chapter 9; shyness and social anxiety, chapter 10; conflict situations, disagreements, anger, and aggression, chapter 11; time management, chapter 12; procrastination, chapter 13; and dealing with basic beliefs, chapter 14).

Bryant and Harvey (2000) warn that psychological debriefing strategies are no substitute for therapy or counseling. When presented alone, or when too much pressure is applied to uncover and share traumatic emotions, problems may actually get worse. Psychological debriefing may be most appropriate as a morale-building, crisis screening, and educational tool. Individuals can be identified who require urgent intervention for dealing with practical health-threatening issues (where to eat, living quarters, where to go for help). In addition, education may ease the process of seeking further and more serious professional help. Such help may include any of the techniques and strategies presented in this text. Of primary importance are:

Exposure, Desensitization, and Stress Inoculation Training

Once in treatment, clients may need additional assistance overcoming and releasing the intense feelings associated with a trauma. Exposure is currently the preferred approach. Through exposure one deliberately sustains imagined involvement in the traumatic event for a prescribed period of time, until intense feelings eventually run their course and dissipate.

Desensitization involves systematically engaging in deep relaxation while fantasizing a stressor, so that distress associated with the stressor is eventually replaced with relaxation. Stress inoculation training involves planning coping and backup strategies for possible relapse. All are covered in chapter 7.

Relaxation

Perhaps the most powerful tool for immediately reducing potentially disruptive arousal is relaxation. Relaxation also enables a client put aside the distractions of the moment, gain perspective, and hopefully find deeper sources of strength and calm. In chapter 4 we consider the most widely used approaches to relaxation and learn how to tailor techniques to individual needs and preferences. In addition, relaxation is presented as more than a tension-relief tool; an important additional goal includes exploring and reinforcing positive personal beliefs and philosophies.

Problem Solving

Traumatic events can disrupt one's ability to solve problems related to a stressor as well as everyday problems in living. Chapter 5 considers useful tools for maintaining a positive problem-solving orientation, properly defining a problem, generating useful alternatives, and selecting and implementing a solution.

Thinking Realistically and Productively

The experience of trauma often elicits negative distorted patterns of thinking, such as viewing the future with chronic pessimism, believing one is completely helpless, and so on. Chapter 6 focuses on how to identify, question, challenge, and replace distorted beliefs with realistic and productive thinking.

Interpersonal Skills

A traumatic event can bring into sharp focus interpersonal coping skill deficiencies, as they relate to coping with both the trauma and life at large. Victims of trauma are often especially receptive to new skill acquisition, including learning how to assertively express one's wants and feelings (chapter 8), listen empathically to others (chapter 9), overcome shyness and social anxiety (chapter 10), and deal with conflict situations (chapter 11).

Task Completion Skills

A traumatic event often presents urgent tasks that must be completed, and important but less urgent tasks that must be pursued later. Deficiencies in time management and patterns of procrastination can have serious negative consequences. Both skills are considered in chapters 12 and 13. More generally, a traumatic event can lead a client to question basic beliefs and values, and pursue such philosophical questions as "Why go on living?" "What is the point of trying or coping?" or "What is the benefit of all of this?" Such basic questions are considered at the conclusion of this book in chapter 14.

ACUTE STRESS DISORDER
AND THE WORLDS OF STRESS

Acute stress disorder is perhaps the purest and most severe form of stress. A pattern of symptoms more severe takes us out of the realm of simple stress into the complex problems of psychopathology and mental disorder. Beyond acute stress disorder are post traumatic stress disorder, mood disorders, anxiety disorders, schizophrenia and psychotic disorders, and so on. Each of these may be complicated by stress, but they involve additional unique properties and call for unique types of treatment. In the chapters to come we consider stress management on its own.

Part II
The Four Pillars of Stress Management

4

ABC Relaxation

Stress management begins with relaxation. Relaxation techniques and strategies are perhaps the most widely applied stress management tools, and the absence of relaxation can itself be a good sign that one is under stress. The present chapter is a guide to ABC Relaxation, a new, psychologically based approach that integrates the diverse rainbow of professional, spiritual, and casual relaxation techniques. First we explore the applications of ABC Relaxation to stress management. We conclude with the concept of *centering* and consider how it is basic to all coping.

First, two major perspectives help us understand how relaxation works: Herbert Benson's (1975) *relaxation response* hypothesis and Smith's (1999a, 1999b, 2001) *ABC Relaxation Theory*. Benson's notions focus on the physiology of relaxation, whereas Smith's theory is psychological. Together, both perspectives provide a balanced perspective of relaxation in body and mind.

Benson has proposed that all approaches to relaxation evoke generalized reduced physiological arousal, a *relaxation response* that is the mirror opposite of the stress arousal response we considered elsewhere (see chapter 2). Instead of increasing, blood pressure, heart rate, breathing rate, muscle tension, and so on decrease. Furthermore, the decrease is deeper than in ordinary casual rest, and is rapid and automatic. One does not have to plan a relaxation response; practicing just about any technique can do it. A refinement of this thinking, the *somatic specificity hypothesis* (Davidson & Schwartz, 1976; Smith, 1999a) proposes that specific body symptoms can respond best to highly targeted relaxation exercises. For example, cold, tense hands might respond to yoga hand stretching exercises; muscle tension in the shoulders might respond to a shoulder massage, and so on.

Benson's relaxation response hypothesis offers a very persuasive justification for learning professional relaxation. Because deep reductions in physiological arousal are the mirror opposite of stress arousal, relaxation can be a direct way of defusing stress and minimizing its destructive impact on health and well-being. Indeed, over 2000 studies have examined the impact of professional relaxation techniques on over 200 problems and concerns. Put differently, we now know that most illnesses are aggravated (and at times caused) by chronic high levels of stress arousal; so it stands to reason that mastering the relaxation response could potentially have a pervasive therapeutic and preventive effect. Professional relaxation methods, the techniques and strategies presented in this book, are very powerful tools, and go far beyond ordinary casual relaxation.

However, Benson's notion of the relaxation response has one serious problem—it suggests that all approaches to relaxation are equally effective and that it doesn't really matter which technique you learn. Although this notion of technique equivalency is unfortunately accepted by most health professionals, research shows it is wrong (Smith, 2001). Different approaches to relaxation have quite different effects, work for different people, and are good for different problems. This became clear when researchers switched their focus from the physiology to the psychology of relaxation.

ABC Relaxation Theory is the first comprehensive psychological approach to relaxation. "ABC" stands for "Attentional Behavioral Cognitive," a summary of what one does in relaxation—focus *Attention* while minimizing overt *Behavior* and mental *Cognition*. In plain English, relaxation involves sustaining the act of simply letting go and simply focusing. This is much more difficult than one might think.

Life is effortful. We strive to achieve our daily goals, anticipate the future, and reflect upon the past. Life is discursive, or ever moving and changing (from the Latin for "moving to and fro"). We plan schedules, vacations, and shopping lists. And when the discursive efforts of life take their toll, wear and tear on body, mind, and soul—we relax. We let go and cease active goal-directed planning, effort, and appraisal. We focus on just one simple thing. *Relaxation is sustained, passive simple focusing.*

Everyone has experienced special moments of sustained passive simple focus. One might gaze at a sunset, and for an instant feel a sense of peace and beauty. Or after reading a moving story, one might close one's eyes and savor the moment, feeling distant and far away from the cares of the world. Throughout life, all of us spontaneously encounter a rich variety of instances of passive simple focus through music, poetry, art, prayer, and so on. Such moments are part of life's treasures; but such moments come and go quickly. The sun sets. The music ends. The poem is finished. We go on with our day's work. The secret of relaxation training is to sustain the moment. This is a very difficult thing to do, like balancing a basketball on a calm and steady fingertip. *Sustaining,* uninterrupted, the state of simply letting go and simply focusing is made easier by practicing a formal relaxation technique. And our research has discovered such sustained focus can have its rewards and surprises.

R-States

The central idea of ABC Relaxation Theory is that relaxation evokes special states of mind, R-States (relaxation states). R-States in turn determine how and when relaxation is effective. This can be summarized in a simple formula:

RELAXATION → R-STATES → BENEFITS

Smith and his colleagues (Smith, 1999a, 2001) had devoted over 10 years to identifying a map of R-States. Research involved over 10,000 subjects and over 40 different approaches to professional and casual relaxation. Research identified 15 basic R-States. The first four represent basic stress relief:

- Sleepiness (Feeling "drowsy, napping")
- Disengagement ("Distant, far away, indifferent")
- Rested/Refreshed
- Energized ("Strengthened, confident")

The next level of three R-States reflects pleasurable feelings one might have as stress is lessened:

- Physical Relaxation ("Physically limp, warm, and heavy")
- At Ease/Peace
- Joy ("Feeling happy, joyful; Having fun.")

Sometimes when practicing relaxation one forgets oneself, personal worries, and concerns, and experiences states that can be described as "selfless." These include:

- Mental Quiet ("Mind is silent, quiet, free of thought")
- Childlike Innocence
- Thankfulness and Love ("Feeling love for others, generally thankful")

At rare moments, spiritual and transcendent feelings can emerge while practicing relaxation techniques:

- Mystery (Sensing the deep mystery of things beyond one's understanding)
- Awe/Wonder
- Prayerful ("Prayerful, spiritual, reverent")
- Timeless/Boundless/Infinite/At One

Finally, one relaxation state simply reflects feelings of increased awareness one may have while practicing relaxation:

- Aware (feeling "Aware, focused, clear.")

These can be organized into a five-level triangular map of R-States (see Figure 4.1).

ABC Relaxation Theory tells us that there is much more to relaxation than reduced arousal. Furthermore, even seemingly ordinary R-States can be precursors to more dramatic states. Once one has mastered the art of feeling R-States Physical Relaxation and At Ease/Peace, other higher states might emerge. Selfless and spiritual states may deepen relaxation and enhance compliance with practice; indeed, when they emerge, they should be incorporated into one's understanding and practice.

Key Indicator R-States

Of the 15 R-States we have considered, extensive research on thousands of individuals (Smith, 2001) indicates three are the best general indicators of overall relaxation: At Ease/Peace, Joy (including feelings of happiness), and Energized (including feelings of strength). An absence of these three states (tapped by the Relaxation Scale in the Smith Stress Management Motivations Inventory) is a good overall indicator of expressed need for relaxation training.

Six Approaches to Relaxation

It is a radical idea that different approaches to relaxation have different effects. Yet this idea is based on a large body of recent research (Smith, 2001). In this book we consider the six approaches to relaxation used most by health professionals and that have the most scientific support. These approaches have quite distinct effects, strengths, and weaknesses. They are:

- Progressive muscle relaxation
- Autogenic training
- Breathing
- Yoga stretching
- Sense imagery
- Meditation.

At this time it is risky to make firm generalizations about which R-States are associated with specific techniques. Our research consistently reveals surprises. It is quite possible that in some circumstances all techniques

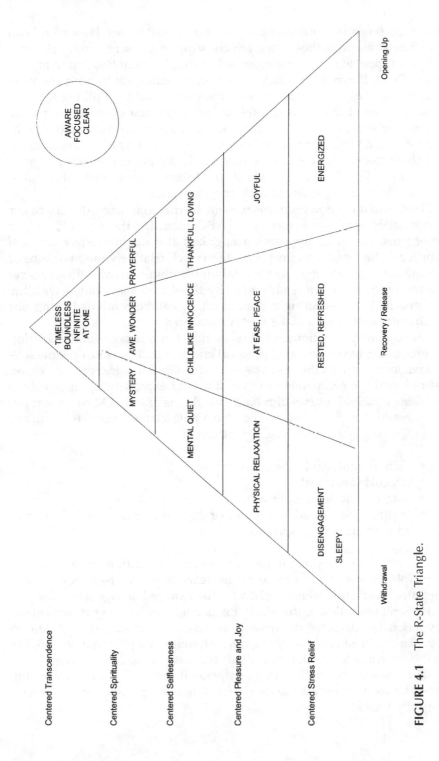

FIGURE 4.1 The R-State Triangle.

have the potential for evoking a wide range of R-States. However, I can venture a few hypotheses, tentatively supported by research. All techniques appear to have some value at evoking Physical Relaxation and At Ease/Peace. Progressive muscle relaxation and autogenic training are physical approaches that appear to be particularly good for evoking R-States Disengagement and Physical Relaxation. Breathing exercises and yoga stretching evoke R-State Energized. Sense imagery is a visualization technique with a broad range of effects, ranging from Physical Relaxation to At Ease/Peace and Joy. And meditation is the simplest approach, one most likely to evoke R-State Mental Quiet, and to some extent spiritual R-States. We will learn the specifics of each approach later.

In the following section we present instructions from the six major approaches from the perspective of ABC relaxation theory. Unlike other programs, the ABC approach recognizes the distinct effect of each approach; therefore, an effort is made to teach relatively pure versions of techniques (breathing alone rather than breathing mixed with imagery) so the practitioner can readily identify the R-States associated with the approach. After mastering techniques, they can be combined using our instructions on how to make a relaxation tape.

First, some precautions about relaxation. On rare occasions relaxation exercises can have unwanted physical effects. While for most people self-relaxation is comfortable and safe, some physical exercises present a level of risk perhaps comparable to that of a mild exercise program, such as walking for 20 minutes or climbing four flights of stairs. Most important, one should stop practicing and consult a physician if he or she has any of the following possible cardiac symptoms:

- Pain or tightness in the chest
- Irregular heartbeat
- Extreme shortness of breath
- Feeling lightheaded, nauseous, or dizzy (these can also be associated with breathing exercises)

Clients under treatment for any medical condition should inform their physicians of the nature of the relaxation exercises they plan to practice. Relaxation training can alter the required dosage levels for prescription medication, particularly for patients undergoing treatment for hypertension, diabetes, depression, anxiety, and any disorder influenced by changes in general metabolic rate. Although the potential for risk has not been consistently demonstrated, the state of relaxation itself is frequently associated with changes in general metabolic rate. As a result, need for medication may decrease (and in a few paradoxical cases temporarily increase).

If a client has any physical symptom associated with a specific organ or muscle group, exercises targeted to this group should generally be avoided (unless part of a properly supervised rehabilitation program). Specifically, this includes pregnancy, injury or recent surgery, weakness, or illness.

Troubleshooting Distractions to Relaxation

Sometimes practitioners experience tension, anxiety, and a variety of distracting thoughts and feelings in relaxation. These are normal and can be an indication that relaxation is working. That is, as one sinks into relaxation, one may become more aware of subtle internal stimuli (such having a belt too tight) and these may be distracting. Also, relaxation can reduce "defensive barriers" we all have to keep unwanted and unpleasant thoughts, feelings, and memories out of mind. Once one is relaxed, these distractions can come to mind. In addition, feelings of sleepiness can be a normal part of relaxation, especially if one needs to sleep. For a careful consideration of negative states that may emerge in relaxation, feelings of sleepiness, and how to deal with such distractions, read *ABC Relaxation Training* (Smith, 1999b), "Troubleshooting," pages 207–213.

SECTION 1: PROGRESSIVE MUSCLE RELAXATION AND AUTOGENIC TRAINING: APPROACHES TO PHYSICAL RELAXATION AND DISENGAGEMENT

Our first set of exercises are primarily physical. Progressive muscle relaxation (PMR) involves actively inducing physical relaxation by tensing up and letting go of various muscle groups; autogenic training (AT) achieves a similar end by passively repeating physically relaxing suggestions. PMR is particularly appropriate for those who have difficulty sustaining attention on a relaxation task (Smith, 1999b); AT is a bit more advanced and requires some focusing ability. Although all techniques appear to have some value for evoking Physical Relaxation and At Ease/Peace, PMR and AT are particularly effective for evoking R-State Physical Relaxation. They are also excellent tools for fostering relaxed Disengagement.

I hypothesize that PMR and AT are most appropriate in situations where deep levels of somatic relaxation are desired. Both may be good choices for dealing with phobias or situational stress or threat in which high levels of somatic tension and anxiety are predominant and prevent one from attempting to cope. In addition, AT may be appropriate for recovering from stress-related medical problems. Elements of AT can be readily integrated with other approaches, except yoga stretching and meditation.

Progressive Muscle Relaxation

Progressive muscle relaxation (also called progressive relaxation and Jacobsonian relaxation) is perhaps the most widely used professional approach to relaxation in America. Early in the 20th century, Edmund Jacobson began work on relaxation as a doctoral student at Harvard, prompted in part by his desire to cure his own insomnia (Jacobson, 1929). Later, at the University of Chicago he conducted research on the knee-jerk reflex evoked by gently thumping an area just below the knee. Jacobson developed a private practice, often making use of relaxation procedures. At first he used reductions in the knee-jerk reflex as a sign of relaxation and a tool for refining techniques. Later he enlisted the aid of scientists at Bell Telephone Laboratory and developed an electronic device for measuring subtle tension-related action potentials from muscle groups and nerves.

Jacobson's original technique involved training clients to detect and recognize increasingly subtle levels of muscle tension and remain relaxed throughout the day. In each session a client would focus on a body part (e.g., the hand), generate the smallest amount of tension possible, and let go.

Most health professionals use a more active form of progressive muscle relaxation, one in which the relaxer first actively tenses up a muscle group (while keeping the rest of the body relaxed), holds the tension for five seconds, and then goes completely limp ("lets go") for 20 to 30 seconds. Those who teach progressive muscle relaxation believe that such initial tensing up creates something of a "rebound effect" which actually enhances letting go and relaxation. Often the image is given of a pendulum. To make a pendulum swing to the right one might simply push it to the right. However, another way is to pull it to the left, and let go so it can swing to the right. Similarly, with progressive muscle relaxation we first tense up (like pulling the pendulum to the right). When we let go, the muscle group initially tensed up automatically "swings" into relaxation. A second reason is to train one to detect often hidden sources of muscle tension. People have considerable muscle tension without even knowing it. Once one can detect when a muscle is tense, he or she can more readily let go and relax.

Instructions

The ABC version of progressive muscle relaxation targets 11 muscle groups. The focus is on practicing relatively "pure" tense-let go exercises in order to identify the specific R-States associated with this approach. It is important to first understand how to tense up and let go of each muscle group. One should study and try the basic instructions below, and then proceed with the actual practice. Remember:

- Tense up for 5–10 seconds; let go for 20–30 seconds.

- The entire exercise should take 25 minutes. If it takes less time, then the exercise is being practiced too rapidly.

I recommend a variation of Goldstein and Rosenbaum's (1982) clever system for pacing this exercise:

- When tensing up, one slowly thinks the word "TENSE" and then spells it out in one's mind by reciting each letter "T . . . E . . . N . . . S . . . E."
- In the relaxation phase, think the words "RELAX, RELAX, RELAX" three times and then mentally spell out the words three times, "R . . . E . . . L . . . A . . . X . . . . . . R . . . E . . . L . . . A . . . X . . . . . . R . . . E . . . L . . . A . . . X." It is important to do this very slowly, so the relaxation phase lasts at least 20 seconds. It is a good idea to first practice repeating the full "RELAX-RELAX-RELAX—R - E - L - A - X—R - E - L - A - X—R - E - L - A - X" sequence a few times to learn to slow down and make sure it takes a full 20–30 seconds. *The most common mistake beginners make is going too fast.* The advantage of repeating these words is that once PMR is mastered, simply thinking the words "RELAX, RELAX, RELAX," or mentally spelling them out, can be used alone as a relaxation technique (especially with a mini-relaxation; see Section 5).

When practicing, one puts a copy of the following list of exercises near by, perhaps posting them on a wall.

TABLE 4.1 Instructions for Progressive Muscle Relaxation

Hand squeeze. Make a tight fist with your right hand. If fingernails dig into your palms, you can make a fist by pressing the fingers flat against the palm, or wrapping fingers around and squeezing the thumb. Let go and go completely limp for about 20 seconds. (Practice twice with right hand and twice with left hand.)

Arm squeeze. Press the lower and upper part of your right arm together, that is, touch your shoulder with your hand. The arm should bend at the elbow. Let go and go completely limp. The hand should fall with a "plop" on one's leg or lap. (Twice with right arm and twice with left arm.)

Arm and side squeeze. Rest both hands in your lap. Press your right arm against the side of the chest, as if squeezing a sponge in the pit of the arm. Let go and go completely limp for about 20 seconds. (Twice with right arm and side, twice with left.)

TABLE 4.1 Instructions for Progressive
Muscle Relaxation *(Continued)*

Back squeeze. Tighten the muscles in the lower back, below the shoulders. There are several ways to do this. You might want to imagine you are scratching an itch, rubbing your back against the back of the chair. Or push the lower back against the chair. Let go and go completely limp for about 20 seconds. (Practice twice.)

Shoulder squeeze. Shrug the shoulders, lifting them up. Let go and go completely limp for about 20 seconds. (Practice twice.)

Back of neck squeeze. Gently tilt the head back, creating a slight squeeze in the muscles in the back of the neck. Let go and go completely limp for about 20 seconds. (Practice twice.)

Face squeeze. Scrunch up the entire face, clenching the jaws, pressing the lips together, tightening up the nose and cheeks, squinting the eyes, and wrinkling the forehead. Everything. Let go and go completely limp for about 20 seconds. Let the muscles smooth out. (Practice twice.)

Front of neck squeeze. Gently tilt the head forward, creating a gentle squeeze in the front of the neck. Let go and go completely limp for about 20 seconds. (Practice twice.)

Stomach and chest squeeze. Gently tighten up the stomach and chest in whatever way feels comfortable—sucking the stomach in, slightly pushing it out, or just tightening it up. Let go and go completely limp for about 20 seconds. (Practice twice.)

Leg squeeze. Pull your right leg back, pressing it against a chair leg, or just tighten it up. Feel the tension all along your leg up through the buttocks. Let go and go completely limp for about 20 seconds. (Twice with right leg, twice with left.)

Foot squeeze. Press your right foot into the floor. Curl your toes and press them down. Let go and go completely limp for about 20 seconds. (Twice with right foot, twice with left.)

Careful examination reveals a certain logic in this sequence of exercises, making them easy to remember. I have found the following visualization exercise remarkably effective in helping clients remember the sequence (it also works for ABC yoga stretching, presented later, which targets the same areas):

We will practice 11 exercises; three focus on the arm, and the remaining eight on the rest of the body. We begin with the arm exercises, which are easy to remember. The first is making a fist, the second is bending the arm at the elbow, and the third, bending the arm at the shoulder. In other words, for the first three exercises we move up from the hand to elbow to shoulder.

The remaining eight exercises are equally logical. Imagine a warm beam of light focused on your lower back, illuminating a circle about the size of a hand. Now, imagine the beam slowly moving up towards your shoulders, up the back of your neck over the top of your head, and down the front of your body to your feet. If the beam travels a straight path—up the back and neck, over the head, and down the front of the body—it will touch each of the body parts to be squeezed and relaxed: back—shoulders—back of neck—face—front of neck—stomach and chest—leg—foot.

For those wishing to make a relaxation tape, read into an audio recorder the instructions in *ABC Relaxation Training: A Practical Guide for Health Professionals* (Smith, 1999b), pages 75–81. Clinicians and trainers should present these verbatim instructions.

One should do PMR twice, once a day for two days, and after the second session fill out the Relaxation Quiz in Table 4.2 (first make six copies!), and score it using the provided key (Figure 4.2). The Relaxation Quiz gives an idea of how this exercise worked in comparison with the other exercises presented here.

Autogenic Training

Autogenic is a popular European approach to relaxation. In the early 1900s, dermatologist Johannes Schultz shifted to neurology and psychiatry and began practicing hypnosis. He made use of the notion that simply thinking of physical sensations can often evoke physical relaxation (Schultz & Luthe, 1959). He then developed an approach to self-directed relaxation and healing, autogenic training, that involved passively repeating suggestions. Traditional autogenic training is a highly structured sequential program (Linden, 1990; Luthe, 1969–1973). Today most practitioners focus on the beginning exercises that involve mentally repeating suggestions targeted to feelings of heaviness, warmth, slow and regular heartbeat, easy breathing, and abdominal warmth—all somatic sensations associated with physiological relaxation and presumably the relaxation response.

It is easy to see the connection between the body and the mind. For example, imagining the taste of a lemon can often evoke the somatic response of salivation. Similarly, thoughts can evoke bodily relaxation. When we relax, we feel physical changes, for example, heaviness, warmth, an evenly beating heart, slow breathing, and so on. Autogenic exercises make use of these feelings. The technique is to simply and passively repeat phrases or images that suggest these relaxation feelings. It is important to do this without effort, or expectation of result. One simply lets words float through the mind like empty echoes.

TABLE 4.2   Relaxation Quiz

[MAKE SIX COPIES OF THIS INVENTORY AND SCORE SHEET]

Relaxation Quiz for (NAME EXERCISE) _____

HOW DID YOU FEEL AFTER PRACTICING YOUR RELAXATION EXERCISE?
PLEASE CHECK ALL THE ITEMS USING THIS KEY.

I EXPERIENCED THIS . . .

① Not at all   ② A Little   ③ Moderately   ④ Very Much

① ② ③ ④	1.	My mind was SILENT and calm (I wasn't thinking about anything).
① ② ③ ④	2.	My muscles felt TIGHT and TENSE (clenched fist or jaws; furrowed brow).
① ② ③ ④	3.	I felt AT PEACE.
① ② ③ ④	4.	I felt DROWSY and SLEEPY.
① ② ③ ④	5.	Things seemed AMAZING, AWESOME, and EXTRAORDINARY.
① ② ③ ④	6.	My muscles were SO RELAXED that they felt LIMP.
① ② ③ ④	7.	I was HAPPY.
① ② ③ ④	8.	I was WORRYING (Troublesome thoughts went through my mind).
① ② ③ ④	9.	I felt AT EASE.
① ② ③ ④	10.	I felt DISTANT and FAR AWAY from my cares and concerns.
① ② ③ ④	11.	I felt ENERGIZED, CONFIDENT, and STRENGTHENED.
① ② ③ ④	12.	I was DOZING OFF or NAPPING.
① ② ③ ④	13.	I felt THANKFUL.
① ② ③ ④	14.	Things seemed TIMELESS, BOUNDLESS, or INFINITE.
① ② ③ ④	15.	I felt IRRITATED or ANGRY.
① ② ③ ④	16.	I felt JOYFUL.
① ② ③ ④	17.	I felt SAD, DEPRESSED, or BLUE.
① ② ③ ④	18.	I felt AWARE, FOCUSED, and CLEAR.
① ② ③ ④	19.	My hands, arms, or legs were SO RELAXED that they felt WARM and HEAVY.
① ② ③ ④	20.	I felt INNOCENT and CHILDLIKE.
① ② ③ ④	21.	My BREATHING was NERVOUS and UNEVEN (or shallow and hurried).
① ② ③ ④	22.	I felt LOVING.
① ② ③ ④	23.	I felt INDIFFERENT and DETACHED from my cares and concerns.
① ② ③ ④	24.	I felt PRAYERFUL or REVERENT.
① ② ③ ④	25.	I felt PHYSICAL DISCOMFORT or PAIN (backaches, headaches, fatigue).
① ② ③ ④	26.	My mind was QUIET and STILL.
① ② ③ ④	27.	I felt ANXIOUS.
① ② ③ ④	28.	I sensed the DEEP MYSTERY of things beyond my understanding.
① ② ③ ④	29.	I felt RESTED and REFRESHED.
① ② ③ ④	30.	I felt CAREFREE.

Exercise: _____

Scale	Scoring Instructions	Score
R-STATE SCALES		
Basic Stress Relief		
Sleepiness	4 + 12 Divided by 2	
Disengagement	10 + 23 Divided by 2	
Rested/Refreshed	29	
Energized	11	
Pleasure and Joy		
Physical Relaxation	6 + 19 Divided by 2	
At Ease/Peace	3 + 9 + 30 Divided by 3	
Joy	7 + 16 Divided by 2	
Selflessness		
Mental Quiet	1 + 26 Divided by 2	
Childlike Innocence	20	
Thankfulness and Love	13 + 22 Divided by 2	
Spirituality and Transcendence		
Mystery	28	
Awe and Wonder	5	
Prayerfulness	24	
Timeless/Boundless/Infinite/At One	14	
Aware		
Aware	18	
STRESS SCALES		
Somatic Stress	2 + 21 + 25 Divided by 3	
Worry	8	
Negative Emotion	15 + 17 + 27	

EXAMPLE. Here is how to score the first scale, "Sleepiness." First add the responses given to items 4 and 12. A person who responded "3" to item 4 and "2" to item 12 would get a total score of "5." Then divide this sum by 2. Five divided by 2 is 2 1/2. Put 2 1/2 in the score box.

FIGURE 4.2   Scoring key for relaxation exercises.

Instructions

Autogenic exercises use passive thinking. A clinician or trainer can demonstrate this idea to a client with the following brief active thinking exercise:

Let your right hand drop to your side. Now, actively and effortfully try to make your hand feel warm and heavy. Work at it. Exert as much effort as you can trying to actively and deliberately will your hand to feel warm and heavy.

Now, simply relax. Let your hand fall limply by your side. Without trying to accomplish anything, simply let the phrase "My hand is warm and heavy" repeat in your mind. Let the words repeat on their own, like an echo. All you have to do is quietly observe the repeating words. Don't try to achieve warmth and heaviness. Just quietly let the words go over and over in your mind. While thinking the words "warm and heavy," you might want to imagine your hand in warm sand, or in the sun, or in a warm bath. Pick an image that feels comfortable, and simple dwell upon it.

Most people find passive repetition more effective.

The autogenic exercises involved here incorporate five suggestions (Linden, 1993):

THINK "HEAVY"

This suggestion is claimed to increase muscle relaxation. A relaxed muscle will actually feel "heavy" because less effort is exerted keeping the muscle firm. A client may notice this when, after an exhausting day, he or she falls heavily into a bed, or becomes so relaxed in a chair that they can barely get up. The instructions are simple: think these phrases: "Feel heavy and relaxed. Hands, arms, and legs feel heavy and relaxed." (Passively repeat over and over, at the same pace "R - E - L - A - X" was repeated for PMR.)

THINK "WARM"

This suggestion is claimed to increase blood flow to the fingers, hands, and feet. When one is relaxed, blood flow increases to the extremities, contributing to feelings of warmth. In contrast, when one is under stress, blood flows away from the extremities, contributing to "cold, clammy hands." Think these phrases: "Feel warm and relaxed. Hands, arms, and legs feel warm and relaxed." (Passively repeat over and over.)

THINK "QUIET, EVEN BEATING HEART"

Most people understand that when they are under stress, the heart starts beating hard, sometimes irregularly. This suggestion fosters a relaxed heartbeat. Think "My heart is beating quiet and even."

THINK "IT BREATHES ME" OR "MY BREATHING IS FREE AND EASY AND EFFORTLESS"

When we are relaxed, breathing is more slow and even. Breathing is both voluntary and involuntary. We can deliberately take in a deep breath. But we continue breathing even when not thinking about it. In this exercise, we simply watch the process of passive, relaxed breathing.

THINK "SUN RAYS STREAMING WARM AND QUIET"

In this suggestion, one focuses on the solar plexus, an important nerve center for internal organs. The solar plexus is halfway between the navel and the lower portion of the sternum in the upper half of the body.

To make an audiotape, read "WEEK 5" instructions in Smith (1999b, pp. 116–125).

Those who do not use a tape should set aside 15 minutes and sit in a relaxing chair with feet flat on the floor. One simply repeats in the mind each of the five suggestions, perhaps thinking of an appropriate supporting visual image for each (warmth—warm sand, sun, or water; heaviness—hands sinking in sand, water). Clinicians and trainers should present the verbatim instructions as published in *ABC Relaxation Training* (Smith, 1999b). After the second practice session, the clients fills out a Relaxation Quiz (Table 4.2, Figure 4.2). This will show how relaxing this exercise was compared with other exercises.

TABLE 4.3   Phrases to Be Mentally Repeated for Autogenic Training

Think "Heavy, heavy, body feels heavy and relaxed. Hands and arms and legs feel heavy and relaxed."

Think "Warm and relaxed. Hands and arms and legs feel warm and relaxed. Like warm sand or water or sun. Warm and relaxed."

Think "My heart is beating quiet and even. Relaxed and even heartbeat. Relaxed and quiet heartbeat."

Think "My breathing is free and easy and effortless. Free and easy. I breathe without trying."

Think "Sun rays streaming warm and quiet. My abdomen is warm and relaxed, comfortable and relaxed."

SECTION 2: BREATHING AND STRETCHING EXERCISES: INCREASING ENERGY

Breathing and stretching exercises are very popular among health professionals and the general public. Although both are often combined, we present them separately because their effects can be somewhat different. Both exercises are very good for evoking R-State Energized (feeling energized, confident, and strengthened), as well as R-State Aware (aware, focused, clear). Like most techniques, both can induce moderate levels of R-States Physical Relaxation and At Ease/Peace. In theory, passive breathing exercises might be expected to induce some feelings of Disengagement, although our research has yet to demonstrate this as a major effect.

I hypothesize that breathing exercises and yoga stretching are appropriate in stress situations where increased energy and confidence are desired (overcoming shyness, becoming more assertive, reducing depression). Because yoga stretching may not induce high levels of R-States Physical Relaxation or Disengagement, it may not be appropriate for countering high levels of anxiety or situational stress. Given the rapid impact of deliberate changes in breathing, and the "portable" nature of such exercises, breathing may be appropriate in situations where rapid, temporary reductions in stress are desired (for example, situations involving anger and provocation as discussed in chapter 11). Breathing exercises can be readily integrated with all other approaches to relaxation.

Breathing Exercises

How we breathe can reflect our level of tension and relaxation. When tense, we often breathe through the chest (notice how boxers and joggers often breathe). When we are relaxed, we breathing is more likely to be diaphragmatic. The diaphragm is a drum-like muscle that separates the lungs from the abdomen. When we are inhaling, the diaphragm moves down, pushing the stomach out; when we are exhaling, the diaphragm relaxes, and moves up into its resting position, pulling the stomach in. As a result, one who breathes diaphragmatically may appear to be breathing in and out through the stomach. With each incoming breath, the stomach extends out, and as air is expelled, the stomach moves in. In addition, relaxed breathing has a special pace: it is often slow, even, and deep (except in very deep relaxation, in which breathing can be shallow). In sum, breathing exercises involve learning to breathe more with the diaphragm, and at a pace that is slow, even, and deep.

Instructions

ABC Training presents instructions for three types of breathing exercises: active breathing stretches, active diaphragmatic breathing, and passive breathing. Basic instructions are as follows (see Table 4.4):

TABLE 4.4 Instructions for Breathing Exercises

Active breathing stretches

Body arch breathing. Make sure you are seated in an upright position. As you inhale, gently lean back, arch, and stretch your back, extending your stomach and chest out slightly. Fill your lungs completely. When you are ready, return to a comfortable upright position while exhaling. Gently tilt your head forward. Repeat the exercise.

Bowing and breathing. Let your arms hang by your sides. Begin to lean back and take in a deep refreshing breath. When you are ready to exhale, sit up. Then slowly exhale as you gently and slowly bow over forward in your chair, letting your chest and head move toward your knees. Let gravity pull you down, squeezing all the air out. When you need to take another breath, pause right where you are, gently breathe in, and continue bowing and breathing out, very smoothly and gently. And when you are ready, begin to sit up, and slowly and gently and very easily breathe in. Repeat the exercise.

Bowing, stretching, and breathing. As you inhale, slowly, smoothly, and gently lean back and gently circle your arms to each side and then to the sky, like the hands of a clock or the wings of a bird. When you are ready to unstretch and exhale, slowly circle your arms down so they hang, and gently bow over, bending at the waist, gently squeezing out the air. Let gravity pull your body down. If you have to breathe out, or in, simply pause, breathe, and resume. Gently sit up, breathe in, and repeat the exercise.

Active diaphragmatic breathing

Stomach squeeze diaphragmatic breathing. Sit up in your chair and open your hands and fingers and place them over your stomach. Spread your fingers comfortably apart so they cover your entire stomach, with your thumbs touching the bottom part of your chest. Now, very easily, take a full breath, filling your stomach and chest completely. And when you are ready to exhale, firmly press in with your hands and fingers, squeezing in, as though you are squeezing the air out of a balloon. And when you are ready to inhale, gradually release your fingers and let your stomach relax and breathe in as if your stomach were filling with air. Repeat.

Stomach touch diaphragmatic breathing. Again, place your hands and fingers over your stomach. As you breathe in, let the air come in on its own, as if it were filling your stomach. Feel the stomach filling, like a large soft balloon, filling completely. When you are ready to exhale, keep your fingers and hands relaxed (do not squeeze). Let the air flow out on its own, gently and slowly. Repeat.

TABLE 4.4   Instructions for Breathing Exercises
(*Continued*)

Passive breathing

   Inhaling through nose. As you breathe in, imagine you are
sniffing a very delicate flower. (Note: a different image can
be selected, like sniffing the waters of a still pond, sniffing
the scent of a candle, etc.) Let the sniffing flow of breath
into your nose be as smooth and gentle as possible, so you
barely rustle a petal. Take a full breath. And relax, letting
yourself breathe out slowly and naturally, without effort.
Continue for 10 breaths.

   Exhaling through lips. Take a slow deep breath and pause.
And breathe out slowly though your lips, as if you were blowing
at a candle flame just enough to make it flicker, but not go
out. (Note: a different image can be selected, like breathing
on a gentle flower, a still pond, etc.) Continue breathing out,
emptying all the air from your stomach and chest. Then breathe
in through your nose. Continue breathing this way making the
stream of air that passes through your lips as you exhale as
smooth and gentle as possible. Let tension flow out with every
breath. Continue for 10 breaths.

   Occasional deep breaths. Let yourself breathe easily and
naturally. When you are ready, take in a full deep breath,
filling your lungs and abdomen with good, refreshing air.
Pause. And when you are ready, relax. And slowly let the air
flow out, very smoothly and gently. And now, just continue
breathing normally for a while. Take three occasional deep
breaths, each followed by five normal breaths.

   Focused breathing. Breathe in a relaxed manner, in and out
through your nose. Try not to force your breathing. Become
fully aware of the air as it rushes in and out, flowing into
and out of your lungs. Calmly focus on the unhurried rhythm of
your breathing. Let yourself breathe effortlessly. Continue for
1 minute.

   To make an audiotape, read instructions in Smith (1999b, pp. 135–146).
Clients who do not use a tape should set aside 20 minutes and sit in a
relaxing chair with feet flat on the floor. Simply practice each breathing
exercise, taking care to move slowly, smoothly, and gently. Clinicians and
trainers should present the verbatim instructions as published in *ABC
Relaxation Training* (Smith, 1999b). One should practice this exercise for 2
days, once a day. After the second practice session, the client fills out the
Relaxation Quiz (Table 4.2, Figure 4.2). This will show how relaxing this
exercise was compared with other exercises.

Yoga Stretching Exercises

Yoga is about 5,000 years old and can trace its roots to ancient Hinduism in India. The exercises presented here are not connected with any religion and represent the safest and easiest of thousands now available. The idea underlying the following yoga exercises is very simple. When we are tense, our muscles are tightened up, like a tightly coiled spring. Yoga stretching involves slowly relaxing muscles through gentle stretching.

Instructions

Each stretch is to be done slowly, smoothly, and gently. It should take about 20 seconds to stretch, and another 20 seconds to unstretch. One should attempt to make each stretch as graceful as possible, not rushed or forced. The most common mistake beginners make is practicing too rapidly, so it is important to time one's first few sessions very carefully, and slow down if any stretch takes less than 20 seconds. We focus on 11 muscle groups, generally the same as those targeted in PMR. A practitioner who has learned the PMR sequence already knows the stretching sequence presented here. One should first read the following instructions and master each stretch before attempting to complete the entire exercise.

TABLE 4.5   Instructions for Yoga Stretching Exercises

Hand stretch. Rest your hands comfortably on your legs (not your lap), just in front of the knees. Focus on the right hand. Slowly, smoothly, and gently open your fingers and easily stretch them back and apart. Try not to stretch so it hurts. Then unstretch. (Do twice for right hand and twice for left hand.)

Arm stretch. Rest your hands comfortably on your legs. Slowly, smoothly, and gently slide your right hand down your leg in front of you. Extend your arm farther and farther like you are reaching to someone in front of you. Reach out and extend your arm, very gracefully, like you are balancing a feather on your hand. And hold the stretch and become aware of the sensations. Then slowly, smoothly, and gently release the stretch. Return your right hand to its resting position. (Do twice for the right hand and twice for the left hand.)

Arm and side stretch. Let both your arms fall limply to your sides. Slowly, smoothly and gently circle your right arm and hand up and away from your body like the hand of a clock or the wing of a bird (Note, select image that works best). Let your arm extend straight to the right side and then circle higher and higher. Let it circle to the sky. And then circle your arm over your head so your hand points to the other side . . . and arch your body as you reach and point farther and farther, like a tree arching in the wind (Note: select

TABLE 4.5　Instructions for Yoga Stretching Exercises
(Continued)

image that works best). Become aware of the invigorating feelings
of stretching. Circle your arm back over your head . . . to
your side. (Twice for the right arm and twice for the left.)

Back stretch. Focus your attention on your back, below your
shoulders. Slowly, smoothly, and gently relax and bow over. Let
your arms hang limply. Let your head fall forward, as you bow
forward farther and farther in your chair. Do not force yourself
to bow over . . . let gravity pull your body toward your knees
. . . farther and farther. It's OK to take a short breath if
you need to. Feel the stretch along the back. Let gravity pull
your body forward, as far as it will go. Then gently and easily
sit up. (Do twice.)

Shoulder stretch. Lift both arms straight ahead in front of
you and let your fingers touch. Slowly, smoothly, and gently
circle them around together, as if you were squeezing a big
pillow. Let your hands cross, pointing in opposite directions.
Squeeze farther and farther, so you can feel a stretch in your
shoulders and back. Hold the stretch. Become aware of the good
sensations of stretching. And gently release the stretch.
Gradually return your arms to your side. (Do twice.)

Back of neck stretch. While sitting erect, let your head
tilt easily toward your chest. Try not to force it down. Simply
let gravity pull your head down. Farther and farther. Focus on
the stretch in the back of your neck. Gently and easily lift
your head until it is again comfortably upright. (Do twice.)

Face stretch. Attend to the muscles of your face. Slowly,
smoothly, and gently open your jaws, mouth, and eyes while
lifting your eyebrows. Open wide. Feel every muscle of your
face stretch more and more. Then gently and easily release the
stretch. Let the muscles smooth out as they relax. (Do twice.)

Front of neck stretch. Let your head tilt, this time backward.
Let gravity pull your head back, but not too far, just enough
to feel the stretch. Do not force it back. Let gravity do the
work for you as it pulls the heavy weight of your head back
farther and farther. Gently and slightly open your mouth, and
let your head relax and fall back. Focus your mind on the front
of the neck stretch as it stretches. Gently hold the stretch.
Then gently and easily lift your head. (Do twice.)

Stomach and chest stretch. Lean back comfortably in your
chair. Slowly, smoothly, and gently arch your stomach and chest
out. Feel a stretch along your torso. Arch and stretch. Then
gently and easily release the stretch. Slowly and easily return
to an upright position. (Do twice.)

Leg stretch. Slowly and easily stretch the right leg out in
front of you. Stretch and twist, so you can feel the muscles

TABLE 4.5 *(Continued)*

pulling. Do this easily and gently. Then gently release the
stretch and return your leg to its original resting position.
(Do this twice for the right leg and twice for the left.)

    Foot stretch. Now focus your attention on your right foot.
While resting your heel on the floor, gently pull your toes
and foot up, as if they were being pulled by strings. Let the
foot and leg stretch more and more. And hold the stretch. Now
easily and gently release the stretch. Return your foot to its
resting position. (Do twice for the right foot and twice for
the left foot.)

To make an audio recording, read instructions in Smith (1999b, pp.
151–179). Clinicians and trainers should present the verbatim instructions as published in *ABC Relaxation Training* (Smith, 1999b). Clients
should practice this 30-minute exercise twice, then complete the
Relaxation Quiz (Table 4.2, Figure 4.2) so comparisons can be made
between techniques.

SECTION 3: SENSE IMAGERY AND MEDITATION—OPENING UP

Sense imagery and meditation are completely mental or cognitive
approaches to relaxation. Although both evoke R-States Physical Relaxation
and At Ease /Peace, they have the potential for evoking much more.
Sense imagery in particular can evoke R-State Joy, and meditation the
R-State Mental Quiet.

    Although sense imagery and meditation, when mastered, have the
potential for evoking sufficient Physical Relaxation and Disengagement
for use in reducing severe anxiety and situational stress, however, these
techniques take time to master. They are perhaps more appropriate as
global preparatory and recovery techniques, exercises to practice at the
beginning of the day to prepare one for activities to come, or recovery
"decompression" exercises at the end of the day (or week) to recover
from experienced pressures and regain perspective. Elements of sense
imagery can be incorporated with all other approaches to relaxation.

Sense Imagery

The ABC approach to sense imagery involves creating in the mind a daydream or fantasy of a relaxing scene or situation. There should be no
effortful goal-directed activity (like playing football, knitting, or engaging

in sex). One remains passive in the image, doing nothing but note relaxing sensations. We evoke four major senses, what is seen, heard, felt against the skin, and smelled. In order to ensure that clients receive the right imagery (without unexpected negative associations), four general categories are illustrated: travel, outdoor/nature, water, and indoor.

Instructions

The practitioner should read these instructions and then practice:

TABLE 4.6 Instructions for Sense Imagery

In our minds we will take a special fantasy journey. We will travel to a relaxing place, far away from the cares of the world, and enjoy what it has to offer.

We now begin our journey.

Imagine you are traveling to a far away and peaceful place. Travel can be very relaxing to many people. In your mind you can move far away from the cares of the day. You might want to think about floating high in the air in a balloon. Can you see the clouds float by? Far below is the world floating past. The relaxing air touches your skin. You can hear the relaxing sound of wind brushing against the balloon. You can smell the clean air around you.

Or you might imagine yourself in a boat floating far out to sea. You can see the distant trees. You can hear the gentle sound of waves lapping against your boat. The water touches your skin. The smell of the water is very peaceful. Your cares are very distant.

Or you might imagine yourself moving through a remote countryside in a train. You can see the pastures rushing past. The creaking sound of the train on the tracks has a soothing quality about it. You smell the wood in the train. You can feel the gentle swaying motion.

For the next minute or so let yourself enjoy a daydream about traveling far away from the concerns of the day. Let yourself become more and more distant. Involve all of your senses. What do you see? What do you hear? What do you feel touching your skin? What do you smell?

[PAUSE 1 MINUTE AND DO THIS FANTASY]

Gently let go of what you are attending to.

We are ready to move on.

In our relaxing journey of the mind, we have now arrived at a distant peaceful outdoor setting. You might picture yourself on the top of a mountain. You can see far into the distance. You can hear the songs of birds echoing. You can feel the crisp mountain air. And the mountain pines smell fresh and relaxing.

TABLE 4.6 *(Continued)*

You might picture a far away grassy plain. Waves of grass extend into the distance. You can hear the wind rushing through the meadow. You can feel the soft grass touching your skin. The peaceful odor of fresh grass fills the air.

Or you might think of a valley. All around are towering mountains. You are next to a giant forest. You can hear the chirping of squirrels. You can feel the warm mountain sun. And you smell the gentle fragrance of flowers.

For the next minute or so let yourself enjoy a daydream about a far away peaceful outdoor setting of your own. Involve all of your senses.

[PAUSE 1 MINUTE AND DO THIS FANTASY]

Gently let go of what you are attending to.
We are ready to move on.
There are many peaceful and relaxing things to enjoy in your relaxing setting. Some may involve the theme of water. What relaxing water setting can you imagine?

You might imagine yourself floating in a pond. You can see deep into the clear blue water. You can feel the water touching your skin and supporting your body. You can hear the splashing of minnows in the distance. You smell the water's clean scent.

Or you might imagine sitting next to a stream. Your feet dangle in the cool rush of water. You can see and hear the water splashing against the rocks. You feel its mist touching your skin. It smells so refreshing.

Or you might picture walking through the mist or rain. Far in the distance you can see the soft clouds overhead. Gentle drops touch your skin. You can hear the rain as it hits the ground. And you notice how clean the rain makes the air smell.

For the next minute or so let yourself enjoy a daydream involving water. Involve all of your senses.

[PAUSE 1 MINUTE AND DO THIS FANTASY]

Gently let go of what you are attending to.
We are ready to move on.
There is more to discover in our special relaxing place. Imagine you discover a special relaxing building or house. It can be anything. You might imagine yourself in a peaceful for-est cabin. You can see the wood walls and fireplace. You can hear the wind outside and crackling fire. You can feel the heat of the fire touching your skin and you can smell the soothing odor of burning logs.

Or you might think of a childhood room. What did it look like? Did you have anything special on the walls. Maybe you can smell food cooking in the distance, or hear pets scampering underfoot. What is touching your skin?

TABLE 4.6   Instructions for Sense Imagery *(Continued)*

Or you might imagine a church or temple, with its majestic and reassuring arches. You can hear the soft sound of music in the background, or smell flowers or incense. As you sit, you can feel the firm chair holding you.

For the next minute or so let yourself enjoy a daydream in a peaceful indoor setting. Involve all of your senses.

[PAUSE 1 MINUTE AND DO THIS FANTASY]

And now, for a moment, think about the journey we have just taken. What part was most relaxing? What part did you enjoy? Did you like traveling? An outdoor nature setting? The water theme? Or the relaxing building or house? Which part of your journey did you enjoy most?

To make an audio recording, read instructions in Smith (1999b, pp. 193–189). After practicing this introductory exercise, one selects an imagery theme, identifies what is seen, heard, felt, and smelled, and then practices for 15 minutes. Clinicians and trainers should present the verbatim instructions as published in *ABC Relaxation Training* (Smith, 1999b). After practicing twice for two days, fill out a Relaxation Quiz (Table 4.2, Figure 4.2).

Meditation

Meditation is a very simple exercise. In fact, the instructions can be said in two sentences: Calmly attend to a simple stimulus. Calmly return your attention after every distraction . . . again and again and again. Although meditation is often associated with religion, the exercises presented here are strictly psychological in nature and not a part of religion.

Instructions

Meditation involves sustaining attention on a very simple stimulus, without thought, analysis, or effort. This can be a frustrating task. Very often the mind wanders and the meditator finds him or herself engaged in thought or fantasy. But this is normal. What is important to remember is that after every distraction, very gently and very easily return attention to the simple focal stimulus. Often one may have to do this many times in a session. That in fact is what meditation is all about.

ABC meditation involves first trying eight meditations. About 1 minute is spent with each. Once a meditation is selected, it is then practiced for about 10 minutes. Start by lighting a candle, which is part of one meditation. Then practice the following sample meditations.

TABLE 4.7 Instructions for Eight Meditations

Premeditation preparation exercises. Before we begin, it is important to let go some of the distracting tensions of the day.

Shrug the shoulders, lifting them up. Let go and go completely limp for about 20 seconds. (Practice twice.)

Gently tilt the head back, creating a slight squeeze in the muscles in the back of the neck. Let go and go completely limp for about 20 seconds. (Practice twice.)

Let your arms hang by your sides. Begin to lean back and take in a deep refreshing breath. When you are ready to exhale, sit up. Then slowly exhale as you gently and slowly bow over in your chair, letting your chest and head move toward your knees. Let gravity pull you down, squeezing all the air out. When you need to take another breath, pause right where you are, gently breathe in, and continue bowing and breathing out, very smoothly and gently. And when you are ready, begin to sit up, and slowly and gently and very easily breathe in. Repeat the exercise.

Let yourself breathe easily and naturally. When you are ready, take in a full deep breath, filling your lungs and abdomen with good, refreshing air. Pause. And when you are ready, relax. And slowly let the air flow out, very smoothly and gently. And now, just continue breathing normally for a while. Take three occasional deep breaths, each followed by five normal breaths.

We are now ready to begin with our tour of eight meditations. We will sample each, and then conclude with the one you liked best.

Body sense meditation. Attend to a physical relaxation sensation you can identify in your body. Do you feel warm? Sinking? Heavy? Perhaps you notice a warm glow in your abdomen. For the next minute or so, simply let go of tension, and quietly attend to that one body sensation. Whenever you start thinking about what you are doing, simply let go of these thoughts, and return to attending to how your relaxing body feels. Close your eyes and try this for a minute.

Rocking meditation. Let yourself begin to rock back and forth in your chair. Let each movement become more and more gentle and easy. Let yourself rock effortlessly. Let your body move on its own, in its own way, at its own speed. All you have to do is simply attend. Let each movement become more and more subtle so that someone watching would barely notice you are rocking. For the next minute or so, quietly attend to gentle and silent rocking. Close your eyes and try this for a minute.

Breathing meditation. Take in a full breath, and relax. Let your breathing continue on its own in a way that is free and easy. There is nothing you have to do. Simply attend to the flow of breath, in and out. And return your attention whenever your mind wanders or is distracted. Close your eyes and try this for a minute.

TABLE 4.7   Instructions for Eight Meditations
(*Continued*)

Mantra meditation. Let a relaxing word, perhaps the *peace*, come to you like an echo in the distance. Let the word go over and over and over, at its own pace and volume. Close your eyes and try this for a minute.

Meditation on a visual image. With your eyes closed, think of the image of a simple spot of light, a candle flame, or a star. Calmly attend. Calmly return after every distraction. Close your eyes and try this for a minute.

Meditation on an external image. Slowly open your eyes halfway. Easily gaze on the candle in front of you. Whenever your mind wanders, gently return. Close your eyes and try this for a minute.

Meditation on sounds. Quietly listen to the sounds that you hear, without dwelling on any particular sound. Close your eyes and try this for a minute.

Mindfulness meditation. And gently let go of what you are attending to. If you wish, open your eyes. The world is alive with sounds and sights and sensations.   You are a mirror. Quietly reflect what passes by. There is no reason to think about anything. With your eyes closed, and without thinking about anything, what do you notice about you? What sound or sight or sensation comes to you? Whenever you notice something, fine. Gently name it, put it aside, and continue attending with an open mind until you notice something else. When you notice something again, just quietly name it, put it aside, and resume attending. Close your eyes and try this for a minute.

- Attending to a relaxing body sensation.
- Gently rocking.
- The flow of breath, in and out.
- Attending to the word "peace" as it goes over and over.
- Attending to a spot of light with your eyes closed.
- A candle flame.
- Sounds floating by.
- Mindfulness.

After sampling eight meditations, one should select which one or two (they can be combined) he or she prefers.

One then practices the chosen meditation for 10 minutes. Clinicians and trainers should present the verbatim instructions as published in *ABC Relaxation Training* (Smith, 1999b). The Relaxation Quiz in Table 4.2, Figure 4.2 should be taken after two practice sessions. To make an audio recording, read the instructions in Smith (1999b, pp. 200–205).

SECTION 4: HOW TO MAKE A RELAXATION RECORDING—ABC RELAXATION SCRIPTING

Over the last two decades, I have introduced relaxation to thousands of students and clients. They have taught me one very unexpected lesson. I used to think that most clients had very specific relaxation preferences and responded best to just one general strategy, whether it was PMR, stretching, meditation, or the like. I spent many years of research attempting to identify the "PMR," "yoga," "meditation," type of person. So far I have found few patterns. All this time, my clients were teaching me something very different; virtually all preferred highly individualized mixtures of many approaches. Very few people prefer just one or two strategies alone.

This discovery has led me to develop a new approach to teaching relaxation, one based on these ideas:

1. Different approaches to relaxation have different effects and work for different people.

2. The best way to teach relaxation is not to impose one or two approaches on everyone, but to introduce a variety of approaches.

3. I try to present relatively "pure" versions of each approach, so that clients can discover its potential unique effects unconfounded by other approaches. For example, I present PMR tense-let go cycles, minimizing breathing and imagery, so clients can clearly note the relaxation effect of tensing up and letting go.

4. Once one is trained in a variety of approaches, we select those that work best and construct an individualized script and tape.

5. The goal of relaxation training goes beyond the relaxation response of lowered arousal. Additional objectives are cultivating appropriate R-States and acquiring beliefs and personal philosophies conducive to deepening relaxation and extending its rewards to all of life.

The analogy of a balanced meal helps explain these ideas:

ABC relaxation is like a balanced meal. Imagine you are at a cafeteria, one with a complete assortment of food. You have decided to forgo the easy temptation to load up on junk food snacks, and eat a truly balanced and nutritious meal. Carefully you examine the major groups of food: vegetables, fruits, breads, meats, dairy products, and so on. You select some from each that you like best, perhaps a little spinach, an apple, a bagel, some chicken, and a slice of Swiss cheese. You end up with a very individualized balanced meal, one you are actually likely to eat and enjoy. ABC relaxation is similar. We learn six basic types of relaxation, the "six basic relaxation food groups," and pick selections from each we like. Then we construct a complete meal from our selections. By doing this we are most likely to achieve a truly balanced "relaxation diet."

Many relaxation instructors present trainees with relaxation tapes, often standardized versions available from various mental health catalogues. However, giving everyone the same tape can pose a variety of problems. Not only does such a strategy ignore client preferences, but it risks exposing trainees to exercises that may have negative associations (see N-States in *ABC Relaxation Theory;* Smith, 1999a). My approach is to craft an individualized relaxation tape based on a mutually-developed verbatim script of exercise instructions. There are several advantages to such script writing:

- The client includes only what works best. (Different exercises work for different people.)
- Different exercises may be selected for a targeted relaxation goal. (Different exercises can be better for different goals.)
- Since the client is inventing his or her own relaxation exercise, he or she is more likely to take it seriously and practice it regularly. Indeed, a client may well treasure his or her script as a truly personal possession, and practice it very seriously.
- Given that training is varied and changing, interest and motivation is maintained, reducing premature quitting.
- Special suggestions and exercises can be included to deepen relaxation.
- Finally, relaxation can be used as a reminder of personal philosophies conducive to living a life of peace and calm.

The Nine Steps for Writing a Relaxation Script

Before starting a script, one first learns each of the six approaches to relaxation presented earlier. (Yes, all six! Remember, relaxation is like a balanced meal.) Then create a script based on exercise elements that worked best. Here is an abbreviated set of instructions:

Step 1. Select relaxation goal
Step 2. Identify R-States consistent with relaxation goal
Step 3. Select specific exercises that work best at evoking desired R-States
Step 4. Arrange exercises and add detailed instructions
Step 5. Incorporate unifying idea
Step 6. Add imagery and meditation details (when relevant)
Step 7. Add deepening R-State words and affirmations
Step 8. Incorporate deepening imagery
Step 9. Add concluding segment

We now consider each.

Step 1: Select Relaxation Goal

One first needs to determine why he or she wants to relax. Extensive research (Smith, 2001) shows that the most popular relaxation goals are:

MEDICAL

Preparing for or recovering from surgery
Managing anxiety over medical/dental procedures
Managing the side effects of prescription medication

SUBSTANCE ABUSE

Controlling tobacco use
Controlling use of illegal substances
Controlling eating problems

PSYCHOLOGICAL DISTRESS

Managing depression
Managing anxiety, worry, and frustration

PHYSICAL DISTRESS

Reducing pain and discomfort
Managing physical symptoms

SLEEP

Dealing with insomnia
Enhancing sleep

INTERPERSONAL STRESS

Dealing with interpersonal conflict
Coping with others

GENERAL HEALTH

Enhancing physical health
Increasing personal strength or stamina
Enhancing resistance to disease

CREATIVITY

Artistic work
Enhancing creativity
Enhancing personal insight

SPIRITUALITY

Spiritual growth
Developing ability to pray
Enhancing ability to meditate

PHYSICAL PERFORMANCE

Enhancing personal alertness and energy
Enhancing sex
Preparing for or recovering from exercise workouts
Enhancing performance at sports

Clinicians and trainers should present this list to the client and ask him or her what his or her relaxation goal is. Record the client's selection on the Relaxation Scripting Worksheet, Table 4.8. See Table 4.9 for an extended example of relaxation scripting.

Step 2: Identify R-States Consistent with Relaxation Goal

At this time, the client will have tried six basic approaches to relaxation, and assessed R-States for each. Now generally familiar with R-States, he or she can take a look at the R-States Triangle (Figure 4.1) and identify which seem most consistent with the relaxation goal selected. For example, if one wants a relaxation script to prepare for going to sleep, R-States Sleepiness, Disengagement (distant/indifferent), and Physical Relaxation might be appropriate. For those desiring to use relaxation as a quick pick-me-up before work, R-States At Ease/Peace and Energized might be more appropriate. Research (Smith, 2001) suggests that a general default sequence appropriate for stress management is:

Disengagement ➔ Physical Relaxation ➔ At Ease/Peace ➔ Energized

Record selections on the Relaxation Scripting Worksheet (Table 4.8)

Step 3: Select Specific Exercises

Once one has learned the six basic approaches presented in this book, the next step is to review them and check which should be included in the script. Summarize scores for each of the six Relaxation Quizzes on the Relaxation Quiz Summary Chart (Figure 4.3, p. 76). These quizzes will reveal which R-States are most associated with each technique. Then select parts of techniques that seem to evoke these states. For example, one might want to experience the R-States Disengagement, Mental Relaxation, Energized, and Aware. Furthermore, he or she may discover that some progressive muscle relaxation, breathing exercises, and imagery evoke these very states. If so, the preferred PMR, breathing, and imagery exercises should be selected. If R-State Sleepiness is evoked by autogenic training, and Sleepiness is not desired, then autogenic training should not be selected. Finally one should avoid exercises that evoke the highest levels of stress. Note that when selecting specific exercises, one does not select an entire sequence, for example, all 11 PRM exercises; instead, one picks parts of exercises that work best. Record selections on the Relaxation Scripting Worksheet.

TABLE 4.8   Relaxation Scripting Worksheet

RELAXATION GOAL:

SELECTED R-STATES:

SELECTION OF SPECIFIC EXERCISES (Which evoke above R-States):

PMR

☐ Hand
☐ Hand and Arm
☐ Arm and Side
☐ Back
☐ Shoulders
☐ Back of Neck
☐ Face
☐ Front of Neck
☐ Stomach and Chest
☐ Legs/Thighs
☐ Feet

BREATHING

☐ Body Arch B.
☐ Bowing and B.
☐ Bowing, Stretching
☐ Stomach Squeeze
☐ Stomach Touch
☐ Inhaling - nose
☐ Exhaling - lips
☐ Deep Breaths
☐ Focused Breathing

IMAGERY

☐ _____
Sights:

Sounds:

Touch sensations:

Fragrances:

AT

☐ Heavy
☐ Warm
☐ Heart
☐ Breathing
☐ Solar Plexus

STRETCHING

☐ Hand
☐ Hand and Arm
☐ Arm and Side
☐ Back
☐ Shoulders
☐ Back of Neck
☐ Face
☐ Front of Neck
☐ Stomach and Chest
☐ Legs/Thighs
☐ Feet

MEDITATION

☐ Body Sense
☐ Rocking
☐ Breathing
☐ Mantra
☐ Visual Image
☐ External Image
☐ Sound
☐ Mindfulness

ORDER OF EXERCISES (from first to last)

TABLE 4.8   Relaxation Scripting Worksheet *(Continued)*

UNIFYING IDEA

DEEPENING WORDS AND AFFIRMATIONS (from Table 4.2 and "Step 7" in text)

DEEPENING IMAGERY

How does imagery begin? (should be relatively active and rich with detail)

How does imagery end? (Should be very passive and simple)

CONCLUDING SEGMENT

TABLE 4.9   Example of Relaxation Script

Step 1: Select Relaxation Goal

RELAXATION GOAL: To reduce stress at the end of the day.
UNIFYING IDEA: The image of a tree bending in the wind.

Step 2: Identify R-States Consistent with Relaxation Goal

Disengagement
Physical Relaxation
Rested/Refreshed
Energized
Joy
Thankfulness and Love
Energized

Step 3. Select Specific Exercises

PMR
   Shoulder squeeze.
   Back of neck squeeze.
   Front of neck squeeze.
AT
   Warm and heavy.
BREATHING
   Exhaling through lips.
YOGA STRETCHING
   Arm and side stretch.
   Back stretch.
IMAGERY
   Tree bending in the wind.
MEDITATION
   Rocking meditation

Step 4: Arrange Exercises and Add Detailed Instructions

Results of the Relaxation Quiz Summary Chart revealed that AT produced the
highest levels of R-State Disengagement, so it is placed first. PMR evoked Physical
Relaxation, so it comes second. Stretching evoked Rested/Refreshed, so it is
placed third. Breathing evoked Energized, so it comes next. Imagery evoked Joy
and Thankfulness and Love, so it follows. Meditation evoked the highest state,
Mental Quiet, so it is placed last.

   Warm and heavy. Feeling warm and heavy. Hands, arms, and legs feeling
      warm and heavy.
   Shoulder squeeze. Shrug the shoulders, lifting them up. Let go and go
      completely limp for about 20 seconds. (Practice twice.)
   Back of neck squeeze. Gently tilt the head back, creating a slight squeeze in
      the muscles in the back of the neck. Let go and go completely limp for
      about 20 seconds. (Practice twice.)

TABLE 4.9　Example of Relaxation Script *(Continued)*

Front of neck squeeze. Gently tilt the head forward, creating a gentle squeeze in the front of the neck. Let go and go completely limp for about 20 seconds. (Practice twice.)

Arm and side stretch. Let both your arms fall limply to your sides. Slowly, smoothly, and gently circle your right arm and hand up and away from your body like the hand of a clock or the wing of a bird. Let your arm extend straight to the right side and then circle higher and higher. Let it circle to the sky. And then circle your arm over your head so your hand points to the other side . . . and arch your body as you reach and point farther and farther, like a tree arching in the wind. Become aware of the invigorating feelings of stretching. Circle your arm back over your head . . . to your side.

Back stretch. Focus your attention on your back, below your shoulders. Slowly, smoothly, and gently relax and bow over. Let your arms hang limply. Let your head fall forward, as you bow forward farther and farther in your chair. Do not force yourself to bow over . . . let gravity pull your body toward your knees . . . farther and farther. It's OK to take a short breath if you need to. Feel the stretch along the back. Let gravity pull your body forward, as far as it will go. Then gently and easily sit up.

Exhaling through lips. Take a slow deep breath and pause. And breathe out slowly though your lips, as if you were blowing at a candle flame just enough to make it flicker, but not go out. Continue breathing out, emptying all the air from your stomach and chest. Then breathe in through your nose. Continue breathing this way making the stream of air that passes through your lips as you exhale as smooth and gentle as possible. Let tension flow out with every breath.

Sense image. The image of a tree quietly bending in the wind.

Meditation. Rocking meditation.

Final Script, Incorporating Steps 5–9

(Note the inclusion of the unifying idea, imagery and meditation details, R-State words and affirmations, deepening imagery, and concluding segment.)

Warm and heavy. You are a tree relaxing in the sun and breeze. [UNIFYING IDEA] Feel warm and heavy, the sun touching you. Hands, arms, and legs feeling warm and heavy. As you relax, you feel distant and far away, indifferent to the world. [R-STATE WORDS]

Shoulder squeeze. A gentle breeze touches the tree. Branches pull together. [UNIFYING IDEA] Shrug the shoulders, lifting them up. Let go and go completely limp for about 20 seconds. (Practice twice; restate in actual script)

Back of neck squeeze. The breeze causes the tree to bend. [UNIFYING IDEA] Gently tilt the head back, creating a slight squeeze in the muscles in the back of the neck. Let go and go completely limp for about 20 seconds. (Practice twice; restate in script.) Let your body feel completely relaxed and limp. [R-STATE WORDS]

Front of neck squeeze. Gently tilt the head forward, creating a gentle squeeze in the front of the neck. Let go and go completely limp for about 20 seconds. (Practice twice; restate in script.)

TABLE 4.9 *(Continued)*

Arm and side stretch. The tree bends in the wind. [UNIFYING IDEA] Let both your arms fall limply to your sides. Slowly, smoothly, and gently circle your right arm and hand up and away from your body like the tree bending in the wind [UNIFYING IDEA]. Let your arm extend straight to the right side and then circle higher and higher. Let it circle to the sky. And then circle your arm over your head so your hand points to the other side . . . and arch your body as you reach and point farther and farther, like a tree arching in the wind. Become aware of the invigorating feelings of stretching. Circle your arm back over your head . . . to your side. Enjoy how you feel more refreshed and relieved [R-STATE WORDS].

Back stretch. Focus your attention on your back, below your shoulders. Slowly, smoothly, and gently relax and bow over. Let your arms hang limply. Let your head fall forward, as you bow forward farther and farther in your chair. Do not force yourself to bow over . . . let gravity pull your body toward your knees . . . farther and farther. It's OK to take a short breath if you need to. Feel the stretch along the back. Let gravity pull your body forward, as far as it will go. Then gently and easily sit up. Enjoy feeling refreshed. [R-STATE WORDS]

Exhaling through lips. Take a slow deep breath and pause. And breathe out slowly though your lips, breathing with the gentle breeze. [UNIFYING IDEA] Continue breathing out, emptying all the air from your stomach and chest. Then breathe in through your nose. Continue breathing this way making the stream of air that passes through your lips as you exhale as smooth and gentle as possible. Let tension flow out with every breath. Breathe in strength and energy. [R-STATE WORDS]

Sense image. Attend to the tree bending in the wind. [UNIFYING IDEA] You can see many trees around you bending back and forth. [DEEPENING IMAGERY: STARTS ACTIVE AND COMPLEX, BECOMES MORE SIMPLE AND PASSIVE] Clouds quickly move past in the sky. You can hear the wind rushing, and the birds singing. The refreshing fragrance of trees fills the air. You can feel the wind touching your skin. The beautiful surroundings fill you with feelings of joy. You feel thankful for this wonderful experience. [R-STATE WORDS] The wind begins to quiet down. [DEEPENING IMAGERY BECOMES MORE SIMPLE AND PASSIVE] The tree bends a bit more gently. The clouds move very slowly. You become more relaxed. The wind becomes a very gentle breeze. [DEEPENING IMAGERY BECOMES MOST SIMPLE AND PASSIVE]

Meditation. Let yourself begin to rock, as the breeze continues. [UNIFYING IDEA] All you are aware of is your gentle rocking. Easily rock back and forth. Gently attend to your rocking motion, back and forth. [NOTE HOW DEEPENING IMAGERY BLENDED INTO MEDITATION] Rock so someone would barely notice you. Let yourself feel very quiet, without thought. Whenever your mind wanders, return to the rocking. Remember, sometimes it is important to let go and take it easy. You can trust the powers within. [AFFIRMATION]

Concluding Segment. Gently let go of what you are attending to. We have completed our relaxation exercise. Slowly open your eyes, letting the light in bit by bit. Take a deep stretch and return to the waking world

	Progressive Muscle Relaxation	Autogenic Training	Breathing	Yoga Stretching	Imagery	Meditation
R-STATE SCALES						
Basic Stress Relief						
Sleepiness						
Disengagement						
Rested/Refreshed						
Energized						
Pleasure and Joy						
Physical Relaxation						
At Ease/Peace						
Joy						
Selflessness						
Mental Quiet						
Childlike Innocence						
Thankfulness and Love						
Spirituality and Transcendence						
Mystery						
Awe and Wonder						
Prayerfulness						
Timeless/Boundless/Infinite/At One						
Aware						
Aware						
STRESS SCALES						
Somatic Stress						
Worry						
Negative Emotion						

FIGURE 4.3   Relaxation Quiz summary chart. Insert the scores for each relaxation quiz in the spaces provided in the table.

Step 4: Arrange Exercises and Add Detailed Instructions

Next decide how to sequence exercises. The default order is that in which exercises are presented in this book. Generally, for purposes of stress management it is a good idea to begin with exercises that foster R-States Disengagement and Physical Relaxation, proceed to exercises that enhance R-States At Ease/Peace, and end with R-States Energized, Aware, Joy, Mental Quiet, and Thankful/Loving. Spiritual R-States (and those higher on the R-State triangle) should be presented later. Again, use the Relaxation Quiz Summary Chart as a guide for selecting which techniques to place first, last, and in the middle of a script. Record on the Relaxation Scripting Worksheet. On a computer, include the complete instructions for each exercise component selected.

Step 5: Incorporate Unifying Idea

The most important part of ABC script writing is selecting a unifying idea. This should be selected and placed on the Relaxation Scripting Worksheet. Traditionally, relaxation exercises are presented in a disconnected fashion, much like workout routines at a health club. In a workout one might do a few pushups, ride the exercycle, complete some situps, lift weights, and so on. Similarly, a relaxation sequence might involve a yoga standing stretch, stretching one's arms, bowing and stretching, and taking a few deep breaths. In ABC Relaxation Training, exercises are woven together so they form a coherent whole, an integrated and meaningful sequence with a beginning, middle, and end. In other words, exercise sequences become something of a work of art. One tool for achieving this is the unifying idea, a statement of a sequence's justification, what it is all about. A unifying idea is an exercise's "title" that explains the gist of an exercise sequence. An exercise sequence with meaning and structure is more likely to be remembered and valued.

For example, in the following segment the unifying idea is "breathing out tension and settling into calm." Notice how this idea is woven into each exercise:

Take in a deep breath. Slowly bow over, let go, and exhale.

Let tension begin to melt and flow out with your breath.

Now we become more calm. While sitting upright, breathe in deeply and slowly and exhale. As you begin to settle into calm, let more and more tension dissolve and float away.

Now, let yourself become even more calm. Let your breathing be effortless and unforced. Simply attend to each incoming and outgoing breath. Let yourself settle into a deeper and deeper-State of relaxation as any remaining tension begins to flow away.

There are many types of unifying ideas. A unifying idea can also be expressed in a simple story, for example, "a leaf floating down the river," "a bubble rising to the surface of the pond," or "the sun dissolving a block of ice into a puddle of water." Here is an example in which such story changes are woven into a sequence of exercises:

Tense and let go. Imagine a bubble is released from the floor of a pond.

Quietly attend to your breathing. Let tension flow with every outgoing breath. As breath flows, the bubble slowly rises.

In your mind's eye simply attend to the bubble as it reaches the surface. It touches the air and bursts, releasing its tension. Let go of remaining feelings of tension.

Here are some more examples of unifying ideas and how they can weave exercise components together:

UNIFYING IDEA: THE RELAXATION GOAL OF PREPARING FOR SLEEP

Tense up your shoulders. Let go. Release some of the tension that keeps you from sinking deeper into a pleasant drowsy state.

Take in a deep breath. Let the air soothe you and calm your tensions. Let the air out, and sink into sleepiness.

Quietly breathe in and out. With each outgoing breath, let yourself become more quiet and drowsy.

Imagine a quiet forest, a dreamlike image as you sink into drowsiness.

UNIFYING IDEA: A PERSONAL RELAXATION PHILOSOPHY, "LET GO OF NEEDLESS CONTROL"

Tense up your shoulders. Notice how this is like trying to control your life. Now relax and let go. Let go of the needless tension you have created.

Take in a deep breath. Hold it in, like you hold in needless tension through the day. Then relax and breathing out, let go of needless tension.

Imagine in your mind a flowing stream. The stream is peaceful, flowing through life without needless control.

UNIFYING IDEA: THE IMAGE OF A BALL OF STRING UNWINDING

Tense up your shoulder muscles. Imagine tension as a tight ball of string.

Then relax and let go. Imagine the ball of string slowly unwinding.

Take in a deep breath. Hold it in. Then relax and breathe out. The ball of string unwinds even more.

UNIFYING IDEA: A PALM TREE BOWING IN THE WIND

Imagine you are a palm tree bowing gently in the wind.

You are on a very peaceful island, far away from any cares and concerns. The wind blows, and subsides.

As the wind begins to blow, tense, let go, and gently stretch.

Stretch farther and farther, feeling a full and comfortable stretch.

And as the wind subsides, gently unstretch, releasing your tension.

As you become more relaxed, attend to the flow of breath.

Imagine a gentle breeze flowing by as you gently breathe in and out.

UNIFYING IDEA: A MODIFIED FRAGMENT OF REINHOLD NEIBUHR'S "SERENITY PRAYER" ("Grant me the serenity to accept things that cannot change, the courage to change things I can, and the wisdom to know the difference. Living one day at a time, enjoying one moment at a time, accepting hardship as the pathway to peace.")

Calmly meditate to the word "peace." Let it float through your mind. "Peace . . . Peace." Tend to that which truly matters.

Gently tense up. Let go, and release the tension. Let go of that which does not matter.

Accept the easy flow of breath, in and out. Attend to the flow of breath. Accept that which cannot change.

It is peace that truly matters.

Breathe gently and easily.

With each breath, think: "Peace . . . peace . . . peace."

In incorporating a unifying idea, it is important to make sure that each exercise element flows easily and logically into the next. Pay attention to the transitions between exercises. For example, the following elements, the shoulder squeeze and deep breathing, are not logically connected and do not flow from one to the next:

Squeeze and release the tension in your shoulders. Let the tension go. Let the tension flow out.

Take a deep breath, filling your lungs and abdomen with air. Then exhale, letting the air out.

Here the same exercises are not only linked by a unifying idea "Let go of tension" but have a transition so that one exercise flows to the next:

Squeeze and release the tension in your shoulders. Let go of tension. Let the tension melt and flow out of your muscles as you let go. With every easy breath let tension flow out [NOTE THIS IS A TRANSITION TO THE NEXT SEGMENT, WHICH EMPHASIZES BREATHING].

Take in a deep breath. Hold the air, then let go, let go of tension, let the air flow out. Let the tensions of the day flow out with the air.

Step 6: Add Imagery and Meditation Details

If sense imagery has been selected to be part of a relaxation, this is the time to elaborate and add details. The same is true if meditation has been selected. Sense imagery should include all the senses (what one sees, hears, feels, and smells) and should be tied in with a unifying idea. Record on the Relaxation Scripting Worksheet.

Step 7: Add Deepening R-State Words and Affirmations

A relaxation script can be enhanced and "spiced up" with words associated with the R-States experienced for each relaxation technique. First, examine the Relaxation Quiz Summary Chart (Figure 4.3) and determine any R-States associated with each technique. Then weave selected words into the script. For example, imagine the R-State word "Energized" has been selected. This can be introduced in a breathing exercise, like this:

"As you take in a deep breath, let yourself feel relaxed and energized."

It takes a bit of judgement to place R-State words appropriately. First, consider which R-States are typically associated with a technique. Then, examining scores summarized on the Relaxation Quiz Summary Chart (Figure 4.3), determine what R-States are actually associated with each technique practiced. Both considerations should help determine where to insert specific R-State words. For example, imagine a practitioner wants to insert the words "feeling far away" somewhere in a script. First, "feeling far away" appears to suggest R-State Disengagement. Disengagement is associated with progressive muscle relaxation, suggesting that this is where the words should appear. In addition, perhaps one's Relaxation Quiz Summary Chart reveals that breathing exercises are associated with the lowest levels of Disengagement, and indeed tend to evoke the opposite R-States, Energized and Aware. If so, one would definitely not place the words "feeling far away" in instructions for breathing.

A relaxation script can be deepened and enhanced if linked with a relaxing philosophy or belief. The most frequent chosen by relaxation practitioners include:

DEEPER PERSPECTIVE

Life has a purpose greater than my personal wants and desires.

There's more to life than my personal concerns and worries.

GOD

God guides, loves, and comforts me.

I put myself in God's hands.

INNER WISDOM

I trust the body's wisdom and healing powers.

There are sources of strength and healing deep within me.

LOVE

It is important to love and respect others.

Treat people with compassion and understanding.

HONESTY

I believe in being direct and clear in what I say, think, and do.

I believe in being honest and open with my feelings.

ACCEPTANCE

I can accept things as they are.

There's no need to try to change what can't be changed.

TAKING IT EASY

Sometimes it is important to simply take it easy.

It is important to know when to stop trying, let go, and relax.

OPTIMISM

I'm optimistic about how well I will deal with current hassles.

I believe in being optimistic.

Generally it is best to incorporate a relaxation affirmation near the end of a script, unless the affirmation itself is the unifying idea.

Step 8: Add Deepening Imagery

Deepening imagery begins relatively active, complex, and discursive (moving to and fro), and then becomes increasingly passive, simple, and focused. We can see this in the following example:

> *You are relaxing on a beach. As you sit up and look around, you notice the blue water and sky. [STARTS WITH AN ACTIVITY, NOT A PASSIVE POSTURE] The sun is directly overhead, its warm rays dissolving tension in your body. You can feel the wind and hear the soothing waves splash against the shore. Birds are everywhere. The sky is full of clouds. [DETAILS ARE COMPLEX AND ENERGIZED] As you become more relaxed, you recline on the beach. The wind dies down to a gentle breeze. Your attention narrows to the sky above and the peaceful clouds floating by. [DETAILS BECOME MORE SIMPLE AND PASSIVE; LESS ENERGIZED] There is nothing you have to think about doing. The air is now completely still. The sky is pure blue and empty. The sea is silent. Simply attend to the sea and nothing else.[MOST SIMPLY FOCUSED AND PASSIVE; LEAST ENERGIZED]*

Structuring an image so it evolves in a direction of increased simple passive focus indirectly suggests deeper relaxation (that is, deeper passive focus).

Step 9: Concluding Segment

When finished with a script, conclude with a "coming out" segment which gently guides a relaxer to let go of what he or she is attending to and return to the everyday "waking world."

Evaluating a Script

Once a script has been written, it is useful to check for possible problems. Are the instructions concrete and specific? Include every detail and leave very little to the imagination. One should not be concerned with filling in missing details or figuring out what ambiguous instructions mean. So instead of saying "Do some yoga stretching with your arm," say "Slowly, smoothly, and gently stretch and reach with your right arm." This instruction is far too vague: "Imagine a cool pond and relax." This one is better: "Picture yourself next to a clear, cool pond. There is barely a ripple. The water is blue. The sky is clear without a cloud. You can feel a calm wind."

One should examine a script for statements that might be questioned. Avoid phrases like:

You will immediately recover from your cold.

You will find the answer to your problem.

Frankly, one may not immediately recover from a cold, find an answer to a problem, or become more relaxed than ever. So avoid making promises that might not be kept.

Similarly, a script-writer should be cautious with absolutistic statements, such as "become completely relaxed," "sink more deeply into relaxation than you have ever sunk before," "you will experience the deepest peace you can imagine at this moment." For some people, such statements can indeed enhance and deepen relaxation. However, others find absolutistic statements worrisome ("What if I'm very relaxed, but not 'completely' relaxed?" "Just how far is 'sinking deeper than I have ever sunk before?'" If problems arise, change absolutistic statements into relative statements that cannot be questioned, "Become *more* relaxed," "Sink *deeper*," "Experience *deep peace*."

One should avoid abruptly introducing exercise elements or images without a previously established context. For example, in the following exercise, the image of a candle flame seems to be arbitrarily introduced:

Your hands feel warm and heavy, warm and heavy.

With every outgoing breath, feel warm and heavy, warm and heavy.

Let your breathing be slow and easy, as your hands become warm and heavy.

Your breathing is slow and easy and relaxed.

Attend to the candle flame in front of you.

Here, the image of a candle flame is given a context.

You are seated by a candle, relaxing in the glowing light it provides.

On your hands, you can feel its warmth.

Your hands feel warm and heavy, warm and heavy.

Let your breathing be slow and easy, so gentle you barely cause the candle flame to flicker.

And your hands feel warm and heavy.

Your breathing is slow and easy and relaxed.

As you attend to the flame in front of you, it burns and flickers freely and effortlessly.

One should be comfortable with the quantity and quality of verbal description you have included. Some people want to be left alone in a relaxation exercise, with relatively little verbal patter. Others prefer to have their exercise filled with patter. Similarly, some are uncomfortable with too much visual and poetic imagery, others prefer it.

How to Make an Audiocassette Tape

One does not have to be an accomplished actor to record a relaxation audiocassette tape. Simply read script instructions into a tape recorder. However, a few guidelines.

- Speak slowly. Most beginning relaxation tape-makers (and a few clinicians who should know better) speak too quickly. I cannot emphasize this point too much.
- Speak softly. (Special professional voicing instructions are in Smith, 1999b). Reading a script is not the same as giving a lecture in a hall without a loudspeaker to a group of elderly who have left their hearing aids at home.
- Most beginners are stingy with pauses and silences. Pauses and silences are essential to relaxation and provide the client with time to complete instructions and enjoy their effects. If one is going to make a mistake, it is better to make pauses and silences too long rather than too short. Few things are more annoying than a rushed relaxation script.

SECTION 5: MINI-RELAXATION

Once a relaxation skill has been learned, it should be applied. Our research suggests that one needs to practice at least five days a week in order to have maximum benefit (Smith, 2001). Most relaxation experts suggest at least a month of practice (Smith, 1999b).

Many active approaches to stress management incorporate brief periods of relaxation lasting one to five minutes. Traditionally, the advice has been to select a cue, such as the word "relax," and consistently think it while engaged in a deep relaxation exercise. Eventually, the cue itself is considered sufficient to evoke relaxation. One simply thinks "relax" when desired (Paul, 1966; Russell & Matthews, 1975).

I prefer tailoring mini-relaxation cues to the individual. First one develops and masters a personalized relaxation sequence, using the scripting instructions presented here. After the complete relaxation protocol has been practiced for a few weeks, the scripting process is repeated. Here, both clinician and client write a mini-relaxation script designed to last from one to five minutes. The mini-relaxation should embody the most effective features of the relaxation protocol already developed.

For example, imagine a student has developed a 30-minute relaxation sequence that incorporates the following exercises with the unifying idea of "Resting on the warm sand by the beach":

PMR Arm and Side (while imagining pushing arms into warm sand)
PMR Back (imagines sinking into sand)
PMR Shoulders (imagines sinking shoulders into sand)
PMR Back of Neck
PMR Front of Neck
AT Warm and Heavy (thinks of body warm and heavy in the sand)
Arm and Side Stretch (stretches in the sand)
Back Stretch (stretches in the sand)
Legs/Thighs Stretch (moves them through the sand)
Feet Stretch (sinks them in the sand)
Deep Breathing (rests quietly in the sand)
Imagery (entertains entire fantasy of resting on the warm sand by the beach)

The first four exercises are presented with numerous suggestions of R-States Physical Relaxation and Disengagement ("Let yourself feel warm and heavy, loose and limp," "Let yourself feel far away from the cares of the day"). The imagery segment concludes with phrases suggesting increased R-State Energized and Rested/Refreshed.

After taping this sequence and practicing it for two weeks, our student decided to make a 3-minute mini-relaxation for use with stress management techniques he was about to learn. In this sequence, he discovered the most powerful components were:

PMR Shoulder
AT Warm and Heavy
Legs/Thighs Stretch
Imagery

All of these are done while fantasizing resting on a warm beach. This became his mini-relaxation. Here is the entire script:

Imagine you are resting on a warm beach in summer. You feel the comfortable rays of the sun on your skin. Squeeze and shrug your shoulders real tight. Squeeze out all the tension. Squeeze further. Then go limp. Let the tension flow out, melted by the warm sun. Let the tension flow into the sandy beach. Let yourself feel limp and heavy, warm and relaxed. And repeat. Tighten up your shoulders. Hold the tension. Then go completely limp, letting the tension flow into the sand. Warm and heavy. Warm and heavy, feeling far away. Distant and far away from the cares and concerns of the world. Relax more and more. As you relax, slowly stretch out your legs and thighs. Stretch your legs out all the way, pushing them through the warm sand. As you stretch, feel the tension sink into the sand brushing against your skin. And slowly, smoothly, and gently release the stretch. Return your legs to a relaxed and comfortable position. Enjoy the feelings of warmth and relaxation you have created, far away from the cares and concerns of the world. In this pleasant state of mind, let yourself enjoy all that you can sense on this beautiful beach: the blue sky above, the soft clouds floating by, the gently waving trees. You can smell the fresh scent of water, and hear the waves gently lapping against the shore. Enjoy this setting with all your senses.

When first practicing, our student made a tape of the script. Soon, he realized he did not need the tape and could do the entire exercise from memory.

I prefer this individualized approach over the traditional cue-controlled approach used in stress management. As you can see, because one is exposed to a wide range of exercises (each with different effects), he or she is much more likely to find exercises that work best. And this individualized process is completed twice, once for completing a full script, and once two weeks later when completing a mini-exercise. One has two opportunities to individualize, vastly increasing the likelihood of selecting a powerful and effective relaxation.

SECTION 6: RELAXATION, CENTERING, AND STRESS MANAGEMENT

Relaxation is the "first pillar" of stress management. At one level, relaxation can limit the destructive impact of the stress arousal response. It can reduce tensions and anxieties that interfere with effective problem-solving. Relaxation can enhance generation of alternative solutions. And relaxation can enable one to evaluate stressful thinking calmly and realistically.

But if we look more closely at relaxation, we see deeper connections. Note that we consider relaxation to be not just a reduction of tension, but fundamentally *sustained passive simple focus*. Given the limited body-based connotations associated with the term "relaxation," let's consider a more psychologically and spiritually encompassing synonym, *centering*. Concretely, both terms mean exactly the same thing, sustaining passive simple focus. We center in PMR by sustaining passive simple focus on tensing and letting go. Centering in AT involves attending to the soothing repetition of a phrase, say, "warm and heavy." For breathing, one centers on the flow of breath, for yoga it is the slow stretch, imagery, the details of an image, and for meditation, the mantra, candle flame, or one's chosen simple stimulus. Each of these is an application of centering, of sustaining passive simple focus in a very direct and concrete way.

But the promise of centering does not end after one has practiced one's chosen exercises, or after one has written a relaxation script or created a mini-relaxation. In the chapters to come we will consider more active ways of centering. To center in action is to do one clear, simple task. It is to clearly know what you want and act—undistracted by unnecessary agendas, distorted thinking, the pressures of others, and so on. This is very much sustained passive simple focus. The simple focus is the task of the moment, what you want to do now. "Passivity" is letting go of needless extraneous worry or activity. And this is "sustained" when one carries a task to completion, that is, actually does what one wants to do.

Each chapter of this book is an essay on a type of active centering. Chapter 5 considers problem-solving, where the centering task is identifying that which one honestly wants, and selecting the most direct and efficient course of action. Chapter 6 considers checking the reality of distorted, irrational, and maladaptive thinking. Such thoughts are enormous energy-wasting distractions to simple action, and learning how to put such thoughts aside is a profound act of centering, of letting go wasted effort and worry. Chapter 7 examines efficient ways of actually putting our best plans to action, of carefully reviewing events and rehearsing skills that may at first seem overwhelming. Once again, this is a centering task, of taking one sustained, simple, focused step at a time, and letting go of extraneous efforts and wasteful indecision. And Part III considers how to live a centered life with others, how to assertively and simply express one's wants, understand the experiences of others, and deal with conflict.

As you proceed with the topics and exercises that follow, it can be useful to keep in mind the underlying importance of centering. The R-States that emerge in the depths of a relaxation practice session are actually signs of centering. Clients may experience these same R-States when they successfully identify true wants, check distorted thinking, and put coping skills to use in daily life. And they will very much experience the R-States of centering as they develop assertive and rewarding relationships with others.

EXERCISES

1. If in a group, each person reads his or her relaxation script. Group members determine how the 9 steps were incorporated.
2. What R-States are associated with different approaches to relaxation?
3. Use the 9-step scripting instructions to create a short, portable 3-minute relaxation exercise you can use in a variety of situations, including at your desk at school or work, at home, or in the library. In selecting exercises, you are limited to two or three. What might be the value of mastering a Mini Relaxation Exercise?
4. Consider each of the major relaxation goals defined in this chapter. Which R-States might be most and least appropriate for each goal? Why? Using results from your own Relaxation Quiz Summary Chart, which techniques might be most and least appropriate for each goal?
5. What relaxation beliefs do you hold? Which do you not believe in? How might certain relaxation beliefs help you practice more regularly, and experience deeper R-States?

5

Problem Solving

We have seen that stress can be defined as wear and tear brought on by perceived threats we can't manage. Another way of saying the same thing is to consider stress as a problem waiting to be solved. This is the perspective of systematic problem-solving, an approach with nearly universal applicability. Although many have offered similar techniques, D'Zurilla, Nezu, and their colleagues (D'Zurilla & Nezu, 1999) have presented the most comprehensive approach.

STEP 1: PRODUCTIVE PROBLEM ORIENTATION

The first step in finding a solution is to consider one's problem orientation. A person who starts with a negative and unproductive outlook is unlikely to benefit from specific problem-solving strategies and their attempts are likely to be doomed to early failure.

There are many self-defeating ways of viewing problems. One may think that problems are somehow "bad," implying mental illness or weakness. Problems may be seen as impossible predicaments. One may blame others, the world, or fate for problems and simply complain rather than attempt a solution. A problem may be viewed as such a significant threat that it must be immediately attacked or avoided, often without first pausing and considering options. One may believe that problems should be quickly resolved and gotten out of the way.

In introducing productive problem-solving orientation, I emphasize the following (Anderson, Reiss, & Hogarty, 1986 ; Bedell & Lennox, 1997; D'Zurilla & Nezu, 1999):

• No matter how dire, bleak, or terrible a problem may seem, there is something, some part of it that can be solved. You may not solve the entire problem today, but at least you can tackle a part of it. And by solving a piece of a problem, you have at least gained practice in assuming a productive problem-solving orientation, and that is a success.

- Problems are a normal part of life, not signs of personal defect.
- Problems are challenges, opportunities for growth and learning.
- Often an acceptable or realistic solution to a problem is not one's first fantasized, idealized choice. "You may get what you need, but not what you first desire."
- Problems take some time and planning to solve; they don't magically go away all at once. It is important to resist the temptation to respond emotionally with the first solution that comes to mind. "Stop and think, and deal with what can be dealt with today."
- Failures can be normal and even desirable. One powerful part of problem-solving is the *trial and error process*. In many learning situations one must first try and fail and try again before getting it right. This is how we learned to walk. No infant ever simply stood up one day and took a power walk around the block. "One has to stumble to learn to walk." It can be useful to view failure as a natural, and perhaps inevitable, part of the trial-and-error process.

STEP 2: INITIAL DISTRESS—IDENTIFYING CLEAR AND CONCRETE PROBLEM CUES

When people describe their problems for the first time, for example to their friends or a stress counselor, they often focus on vague and global feelings of distress. One might hear:

"My problem is that I feel overwhelmed and helpless."

"I'm feeling so down and out of it. Things are all going wrong."

Even when a relatively specific problem situation is alluded to, the focus is still often vague and primarily centered on distress:

"My spouse and I argue. I'm so frustrated I just don't know what to do."

"I just can't seem to make ends meet. Everything is so up in the air. I don't know if I can ever make it."

Step 2 in problem-solving involves expressing such initial distress, and then clarifying it in terms that are concrete and specific. For example, an initial vague statement of distress, "I'm so frustrated," might be concretely and specifically clarified, "I'm so frustrated. I'm very angry at my spouse, but don't know why." Note the vague feeling of "frustration" is now a feeling of "anger."

Such a process of clearly stating distress sets the stage for later problem-solving. For example, consider the kinds of problems a physician might encounter. If you were a physician treating a patient, you would want your patient to see you early, when symptoms first emerged, and you would want clear information about what the symptoms were. It would not be helpful for a patient to report:

> "Oh, I'm having some sort of a breathing problem. It's been going on for a few weeks. Sometimes I sneeze. It's hard for me to breathe. I don't feel well. I feel sort of out of it all over. Sort of nervous and upset."

It would be better for a patient to give symptom information that is early, clear, and concrete, like this:

> "My head is congested, and I have been coughing frequently. It is hard for me to breathe. Sometimes my nose is entirely blocked. I have a fever and my muscles ache. I feel warm and am perspiring. I seem to lack energy and can't climb a flight of stairs without getting out of breath."

These symptoms are very clear, concrete, and timely. They help point the physician in the direction of a correct diagnosis of the problem, perhaps the flu, bronchitis, or even pneumonia. Given that the symptoms were caught early, treatment is more likely to succeed.

Most problem-solving experts (for example, Bedell & Lennox, 1997 and D'Zurilla & Nezu, 1999) recommend looking at three types of distress: thoughts, behaviors, and feelings. *Distressed thoughts* include negative and distorted ideas about a problem and oneself. Client reports of excessive worry, obsessive rumination, "can't get negative thoughts out of mind" are excellent indicators of underlying distorted thinking. It is easy to get caught up in thought symptoms and mistake them for the true problem. We can see such misattribution in the following examples:

> "Nothing is going right for me. This is the end of the world. This is a catastrophe. That's my problem."

> "I just go over and over my financial plight in my mind. I can't stop thinking about it. Somehow I think things will get better if I just keep thinking about it. I get a false sense of control."

> "Everyone should have a perfect lover. And I'm all alone. I feel so isolated. What a problem!"

In none of these examples do we really know what the real, underlying problem is. In the following examples, each of these thoughts is identified as a warning sign that there is a problem that needs to be solved.

"Nothing is going right for me. This is the end of the world. I am helpless. Now, wait. Whenever I get caught up in this type of thinking, I'm spinning my wheels and getting nowhere. I think this way when there's a problem that needs to be solved."

"I just go over and over my financial plight in my mind. I can't stop thinking about it. I now know this obsessing is a sign that something's wrong. There's some business I need to tend to. It doesn't help to get preoccupied with worry. Let's get to the real problem."

"I think everyone should have a perfect lover. That's nonsense! In the real world many people have friends, not lovers, and some are relatively alone. OK, this type of thinking is getting me nowhere. But it sure lets me know that I've got some sort of problem that needs attention."

Sometimes *distressed behaviors* serve as cues that something is wrong and a problem exists. This is particularly true if the behavior is unusual for a person (staying away from work, avoiding certain people, compulsively engaging in escapist activities, drinking), self-destructive, or potentially destructive to others. In addition, persistent mistakes and coping failures can be signs of a problem ("whenever I try to meet someone new, they walk away.") Again, one can become preoccupied with the symptom (and never solve the underlying problem), or see the symptom as a cue that action needs to be taken.

People often label *negative feelings* as the "real problem." However, such feelings as anxiety, depression, anger, and the like are emotional consequences of problems. Generally, a negative feeling is most likely to signify an underlying problem if it is particularly intense, frequent, long-lasting, and inappropriate to the situation (Bedell & Lennox, 1997). Most important, problem-feelings are often initially vague and fuzzy ("I feel upset, bad, messed up, unhappy") or global and all-inclusive without a clear referent ("I hate my husband, I'm depressed about my life, everything makes me so tense and nervous.")

I suggest two ways of identifying and clarifying distressed feelings; one is analytic and one nonanalytic.

Analytic Cue Clarification

An analytic approach starts with the idea we introduced in chapter 2 that emotional distress involves three basic categories of feelings (Plutchik, 1994): anxiety, depression, and anger. Sometimes an individual may be distressed and confused because they experience combinations of these negative emotions. For example, a mother may be both angry and sad that her son skipped school; she may be confused by this mix of feelings.

Often one is simply aware of only the somatic or bodily component of a feeling, having tuned out the emotional component. The husband of the son who skipped school may suddenly have an unexplained stomachache, and not be aware of his underlying anger. And feelings can be "fuzzy" or imprecise. One might feel "bad, messed up, upset, crazy, awful, etc."

An analytic way of approaching such feelings would consider the following:

> Experts suggest that many negative feelings can fall into three categories: Fear and anxiety, sadness, and anger. For example, if you feel fear and anxiety, you may feel worried, terrified, dread, and fright. A sad person may feel hopeless, depressed, discouraged, unhappy. An angry person may feel irritation, annoyance, bitterness, insulted. Which of these basic four feelings seems to best fit what you are feeling?

There is a value in identifying which of the three categories a feeling reflects. Each category is often associated with different thoughts and behaviors (Bedell & Lennox, 1997). For example, the dictionary tells us that fear and anxiety are associated with the expectation that something bad and unwanted has happened or will happen. It is often associated with avoidance behavior and denial (fleeing the threat). Sadness is associated with wanting something, not getting it, and giving up hope. A sad individual displays inactivity, withdrawal, lack of interest, and so on. Anger is associated with frustration and destructive or attacking behavior or speech. Awareness of these links can help clarify cues that a problem exists and what it is. Armed with this information, one can offer or consider an interpretation of a vague distressed feeling:

DISTRESSED PERSON:	"I feel really out of it. It was important that my spouse recognize my phone call as a way of expressing my love. I don't feel like doing anything."
CLARIFYING INTERPRETATION:	"I sense you feel a little blue or depressed that your spouse didn't recognize your expression of love."

Nonanalytic Cue Clarification

Sometimes thinking too much about a problem makes it worse. An alternative way of clarifying problem cues involves ceasing analytic thought. This can be applied most directly to clarifying one's wants and feelings, and perhaps somewhat less so to associated cue behaviors.

We will consider the process of "focusing" introduced by Eugene Gendlin (1981). One should not confuse this conceptualization of focusing with the notion of focusing associated with relaxation in chapter 4; "Gendlin's focusing" refers to a technique for clarifying cues; "Smith's focusing" is a relaxation skill for attending to a simple, relaxing stimulus. Here are the steps I use (Smith, 1993b) when teaching Gendlin's focusing:

Step 1: Clear a Space

Focusing is not the same as actively trying to analyze or figure out a problem. In fact, the first step is to put such efforts aside and take a break from all analytic thought. One will have plenty of time to figure out problems later; now is the time to take a rest and create a mental space. Practicing a relaxation exercise can help in this process of "clearing a space" (chapter 4).

Step 2: Attend to the Gut Problem Feeling or Want

The first sign of stress people feel is often a vague feeling of discomfort. For example, you may have just finished a shopping trip to the mall. You stop because something feels wrong. You aren't sure what it is, but you have a vague sense you have forgotten something. A few ideas come to mind. "I forgot to feed the dog. No, that's not it. I forgot to water the plants. No. This is it, I forgot to go to the shoe store. I was planning on purchasing some shoes." Such "something is wrong" feelings are vague and fuzzy, and include:

"Deep down inside I feel afraid for some reason."

"I'm confused and have no idea why."

"Why am I so anxious? What could possibly be wrong?"

"I feel guilty, but I can't identify anything I've done."

"I feel blue and down. Just blue and down, for no apparent reason."

"My life feels empty and incomplete. Why?"

These vague feelings are very important in defining the starting point of the focusing exercise. Gendlin explains they can be the tip of an iceberg, the very surface of very important underlying thoughts and emotions. The first step in uncovering what is hidden is asking a simple question.

Step 3: What Is the "Gist," the "Crux" of the Gut Problem Feeling?

It is important not to try to push the feeling away or solve it. Instead, one asks "What is the gist or crux of the felt problem?" And simply wait. If your mind wanders, that is OK. Simply return attention to attending to the gut problem feeling, not any particular thought.

Step 4: The "zig-zag-A-hah" Process

Continue attending to what is felt as the gist or crux of a problem, without trying to figure it out or label it. As one attends, many thoughts and feelings may come and go. But just wait, without deliberately picking or analyzing anything that comes to mind. It is as if one were watching leaves float by on a stream. Attend to what comes and goes. In time, a special word or image might emerge that fits the feeling perfectly. How does one know it fits? It simply feels right; one might even have a small "ah-ha" insight experience.

Step 5: Attend to the New Gut Feeling

The original feeling may now open up slightly, become more clear. You may understand more of it. Here you have a choice—repeat the process on the new gut feeling (waiting for the "crux," and so on), or simply stop.

Gendlin's focusing exercise can be readily applied to stress problems that seem resistant to change. If one is confused about what his or her real problem is, it can be useful to focus on that very feeling of distress, whatever it may be. We can see this process in the following example:

> I feel vaguely upset and don't know why. I just feel bad. I've tried to figure out my negative feeling, but without success. I even tried to think positive and get involved in positive activities, but the feeling remained. Then I stopped, put my thinking aside, and just attended to my negative feeling. It was a dark feeling in my gut. I passively attended to it and asked, "What is the gist, the most important thing about this feeling?" Then I waited. Sometimes thoughts came and went, like "I did something wrong to my wife," "I paid too much for my car," or "I spoke harshly to my child." None of these thoughts felt right. I continued attending. Then, the thought came up, "I'm trapped at work. I feel like I'm in a dungeon at work. A dungeon." That was right. A veil lifted, I took a little breath and sighed. My vague negative feeling had changed, or opened up into another feeling, "feeling trapped and hopeless." I kept at it, and attended to the dungeon feeling. Many thoughts came and went, until another felt just right, "I'm going nowhere. I have no future here. I'm trained to do much more, and I'm stuck at a job that just isn't satisfying to me." That was it.

In this example we can see all steps of the focusing exercise. The initial vague feeling was "I just feel bad." As long as our person quietly and nonanalytically attended to this nonverbal feeling, thoughts came and went until one emerged that articulated an underlying feeling, "I feel trapped." This too is a feeling, one a bit more focused than "feeling bad." Our person attended to it, and one other feeling emerged, even more precise, "I have no future in my job."

Summary

Once one has expressed vague feelings of distress, he or she is ready to identify clear and concrete distressed thoughts, behaviors, and feelings. This is part of the initial problem-solving process of fully expressing distress. In summary, this process serves two functions:

1. Early warning cues are identified that something is wrong and problem-solving action should be taken.
2. Clear and specific symptoms help point a client in the direction of getting to the true source of a problem, much as clear and specific symptoms help a physician make accurate diagnoses.

STEP 3: DEFINING THE PROBLEM IN A WAY MOST LIKELY TO BE SOLVED

"A well-defined problem is half-solved" (D'Zurilla & Nezu, 1999). Once one has identified that a problem exists, it needs to be defined in a way that can be solved.

Define a Specific Problem Situation: The "Four W's"

Vague, emotional problems are difficult to solve; problems defined in terms of a specific "defining situation" are better. It is not likely that one can solve an entire complex problem immediately; indeed that is not how most problems in life are resolved. It is better to focus on a piece of the problem that is most solvable now, a piece that can be identified in terms of a specific, concrete situation or event.

After a problem has been identified, one gathers concrete information, much as a police detective would gather the facts at a crime scene, or a news reporter gather details for a story. Often, problem-solving experts recommend focusing on four "W's" in gathering information: *When* did this happen? *Where* were you? *Who* was there? *What* did you and others do, say, think, and feel? To this we can add what might be the most important "W," what did you *Want?*

What Do You Want in This Situation? The "How Can I"

As one identifies a specific want in the problem situation or event, it is important to phrase it as a positive "how can I" statement (Bedell & Lennox, 1997). Such a statement expresses one's want not in terms of getting rid of something, but in terms of getting something. For example, one might say "How can I improve my work conditions" rather than "I want to get rid of the bad conditions at work."

Many clients have difficulties at the stage of problem definition. If a problem is poorly defined, it is unlikely to be solved. One can increase the likelihood that the right problem has been defined by asking three questions:

1. Is there a subgoal I need to address first before I can act on my "to do statement"? If so, this should be made the goal.
2. Is what I want to do actually within my power to achieve?
3. Is my "how can I" phrased in a positive way?

Often, it is useful to list five to ten goals and subgoals for one's concrete problem situation, and then select the one that is most solvable at the present moment.

STEP 4: GENERATING ALTERNATIVE SOLUTIONS

After a problem has been clearly defined, the next step is to consider solutions. People under stress often use the first solution that comes to mind, or complain of a lack of solutions. Brainstorming is an effective way of maximizing the likelihood that a good solution will be found.

Brainstorming involves putting aside inhibitions and generating as many potential solutions as one can think of. The principle is that reducing constraints can enhance the likelihood that one will think of ideas, and that producing many ideas enhances the likelihood of finding one that works. When brainstorming, it is important to temporarily put aside critical thinking, and let the imagination run free. Silly, inappropriate, or ridiculous ideas are fine. In addition, the greater the variety of ideas the better. It is important not to fall into an "idea rut" and think of ideas of only one type. One thinks of broad strategies (To make money one might "get a job," "win a contest," or "find a very rich mate") or very specific tactics that are part of more general strategies ("To find a job, look in the newspaper and the Web, and ask friends"). It can be useful to change one's frame of reference, and imagine how someone else (a respected friend) might brainstorm answers. A variation of this approach involves using imagery (chapter 4) to visualize encountering a problem and coming up with solutions. In addition, one might identify similar problems successfully confronted in the past, and borrow solutions ("How can I find a job? Last year I found a new apartment by asking my relatives and friends for ideas. I could try that now and ask them for job ideas.")

Generally, these strategies enable one to consider a greater diversity of *categories* of possible solutions. One way of enhancing category diversity is to sort an initial listing into groups reflecting similar categories. One then determines a title for each category grouping. For example, a client might brainstorm solutions to the question "What are some of the unusual uses one might have for used bubble gum?" An initial brainstormed list might include:

> Make the gum a work of art
> Build a dollhouse out of several globs of gum
> Flatten gum out into a pavement for walking
> Build a house for fish
> Make a gum doggie
> Use gum to stick pebbles together for a tower
> Make a sidewalk out of gum
> Build a gum bridge
> Make a gum person ("gumbo")
> Make a sculpture
> Create a gum worm for fishing.

These could be sorted into the following categories:

> Creative
>   A work of art
>   A sculpture
> Buildings
>   Dollhouse
>   House for fish
>   Tower
> Pathway
>   Pavement
>   Sidewalk
>   Bridge over an aquarium
> Living things
>   A person
>   Gum doggie
>   A gum worm

After doing this, brainstorming is continued in which one thinks of both additional solutions and additional categories.

STEP 5: MAKING THE DECISION

Brainstorming can produce a wealth of ideas, some good and some not so good. The obvious next step is to evaluate the ideas generated and select the one to implement. First weed out the solutions that are obviously inappropriate. Then, evaluate the remaining plausible options using these criteria.

1. Does the option under consideration actually get what I want (as specified in my "How can I" statement)? Here one reconsiders one's definition of the problem, STEP 3, and determines if each solution actually solves the problem.
2. Does it require first achieving one or more subgoals? If so, the subgoal and its solution should again be addressed. For example, imagine one's goal is "To find a job." It becomes clear that first one has to find some list of job possibilities. A subgoal might be "To find a list of job opportunities." A further subgoal here might then be "To find which newspapers have good job listings." The problem and solution then have been refined from "to find a job" to "to find newspapers with job listings."

Solutions that survive the above two criteria can be evaluated with the following secondary criteria (Anderson, Reiss, & Hogarty, 1986 ; Bedell & Lennox, 1997; D'Zurilla & Nezu, 1999), some already used to evaluate wants (STEP 3).

1. Are there no serious obstacles to implementing this solution? If there are obstacles, what are they?
2. Is the solution within my capacity and resources (financial, time available, effort required)? Generally, do not state a goal that requires someone else to fulfill ("I want my wife to clean the dishes").
3. Is the solution legal, socially acceptable, and not going to violate the rights and feelings of others?
4. Does this solution have a reasonable back-up contingency plan if my first choice doesn't work?
5. Will I learn or gain something if this solution doesn't succeed in getting the want I specify? Increased self-esteem? Practice in solving problems?

One simple way of using these criteria is to compute a score for each solution. Each criterion is worth one point. A solution that meets all five criteria gets a score of 5, a solution that meets only the first and fourth criteria gets a score of 2.

Finally, one selects the solution with the highest score. A decision is made whether to attempt the solution or not. If unsure, one can complete a "cost/benefit analysis" and simply list in one column all of the benefits of attempting this solution, and in a second column all of the costs. Once these are listed, one decides again whether the solution is worth trying.

STEP 6: TAKING ACTION:
CUE–RESPONSE–CONSEQUENCE

Good plans are useless unless actually attempted. If a client procrastinates or can't find time to put a plan into action, consider later chapters on time management and procrastination (chapters 12 and 13).

A clinician may make an action contract with a client. Such a contract includes three parts:

1. The *cue*, or signal that indicates precisely when to deploy one's plan.
2. The *response*, or actions one has agreed to try.
3. The *consequence*, or simple reward (like a pat on the back, self-congratulation, ice cream cone, or other treat) and honest evaluation of what worked, what didn't work, what might be tried in the future, and most important, what was learned. If a problem-solving plan does not work, a previously identified backup plan is the appropriate next step. Or a newly uncovered obstacle becomes the problem-to-be-solved. Or, having gathered new information through actually trying a solution, one can start the problem-solving process over with STEP 1. Most important, in problem-solving, there are no absolute failures, just steps to finding the best goal and best solution.

This simple formula, Cue–Response–Consequence, is an apt summary of our chapter on problem-solving. It will serve as a guiding idea for chapters to come.

EXERCISES

1. Imagine you are trying to illustrate the productive problem-solving orientation to someone else. Think of an example in your own life that reflects each of the listed six characteristics of the productive problem-solving orientation (STEP 1). Explain how each is illustrated.

2. Think of a problem you had this month. Construct two definitions, one that meets and one that does not meet the criteria presented in the text.

3. Consider a problem you recently experienced. What emotions did you have? Can your emotions be understood in terms of "fear, anger, or anxiety?"

4. Consider a problem you experienced in which your feelings were confused or not clear. Was your inclination to (1) flee, avoid, or deny, (2) attack or confront, or (3) give up? According to your text, what emotion is often associated with each? What emotions did you experience?

5. Try Gendlin's focusing exercise. Describe what parts worked or didn't work.

6. Select a relaxation exercise to practice before Gendlin's focusing exercise. What did you select, and why? Did it work?

7. Think of a problem in your own life in which a productive problem-solving orientation was not displayed, and the problem was aggravated. Identify which of the characteristics was absent.

8. Select a problem in your life. What was your original definition, before reading this book? Define the problem again using the criteria in STEP 3. What was missing (if anything) in your original definition?

9. Ask someone you know to define a recent problem in their life. What problem-defining criteria did they display? What criteria did they not use? How did their definition contribute to or interfere with actually coming up with a workable solution?

10. Brainstorming involves suspending critical thinking and generating many possible solutions. Brainstorm as many solutions as you can to this problem:

> You are the president of a toy company that manufactures small female figures similar to the famous "Barbie Doll." Unfortunately, your plant has just produced 50,000 dolls with one defect—-they were missing their hair. You have only a week to sell these dolls, not enough time to manufacture a new set, or sew hair on. Think of all of the potential uses you can for hairless dolls.

Sort your solutions into categories. Name each category. Identify any strategies or tactics. Resume brainstorming.

11. Brainstorm solutions to this problem:

> You are on a TV game show, "The Billionaire Brainstorm Show," and your question is: Think of all of the unusual (and usual) uses you can for spoons. You may alter your spoon(s) in any way you wish.

Sort your solutions into categories, and continue brainstorming. Evaluate the 5 best brainstormed solutions according to each criterion in your text.

12. Think of a recent problem. After defining your want, brainstorm possible solutions. Sort your brainstormed solutions into categories, and identify which are tactics and which are strategies. Then resume brainstorming.

13. Evaluate the five best brainstormed solutions according to each criterion in your text. Give each a score using the decision-making criteria in STEP 5.

14. Those who have difficulty with problem-solving often display a type of distorted thinking called "Childlike Fantasy" in which one assumes (as children may do) that everything should go one's way. People displaying Childlike Fantasy may think such things as "everyone should be nice and love each other" and "problems should have happy endings." Discuss why Childlike Fantasy may interfere with each step of effective problem-solving.

15. In what ways can problem-solving be a centered activity, involving letting go and simple, sustained focus? Include the role of R-States.

6

Thinking Realistically and Productively: The Smith Irrational Beliefs Inventory

Popular culture often promotes the importance of cognitions, that is, thoughts, beliefs, perceptions, attitudes, in determining or aggravating stress. We can see this in truisms ("it's all in the mind") and a burgeoning library of self-help books. However, popular considerations of cognition are often oversimplified and easily discounted. In this chapter we consider how distorted thinking can create stress, and the many ways distorted thinking can be converted to realistic and productive thinking. We begin with an example:

> Bea and Betty are young adults who have broken up with their first boyfriends (after 6 months of dating). However, Bea is under substantial stress, whereas Betty is not. Bea is depressed, withdrawn, and suffers from headaches. She risks her job by taking an abundance of "mental health holidays" and is letting her college grades slide. Betty is also sad and frustrated. However, she still gets together with her friends and has little difficulty continuing with work and school. Given that Bea and Betty have experienced the same stress event, why are they reacting so differently? The answer is in their thoughts. Bea frequently worries: "I will never date another man. I'm going to live my life alone. No one will ever like me." However, Betty's thoughts are a bit different: "Sure, it's a big frustration. However, it isn't the end of the world. I still have my friends, job, and school. And this breakup can teach me something about dating guys in the future."

Identical stress situations can be rendered stressful or benign depending on our thoughts or appraisals. Bea's thoughts about her breakup with her boyfriend ("I will never date another man. I'm going to live my life alone. No one will ever like me.") turn a simple frustration and disappointment into a very severe problem, one of disastrous proportions. And because her thinking precludes the possibility of finding other dates, finding satisfaction with friends, or being liked, a solution is difficult to envision. No wonder Bea is withdrawn and depressed. However, Betty honestly recognizes a frustration for what it is (bad but not a disaster) and does not preclude the possibility of finding solutions (learning from this experience).

SECTION 1: UNDERSTANDING THE ROLE OF DISTORTED THINKING

Albert Ellis (1962), one of the founders of cognitive therapy and an early stress pioneer, has suggested a formula for the relationship between emotions and cognitions, the "A-B-C model" (not to be confused with my ABC Relaxation Theory, presented in chapter 4). Because of its nearly universal application in the field of stress management, I will note it here; however, we will use a slightly different schema. According to Ellis, most people think in simple stimulus-response terms, that external events cause negative distressing emotions or symptoms; as Ellis would put it, Activating events or cues ("A") cause emotional/symptomatic Consequences ("C"). For example, one might think:

"My boss rejected my report (A) and made me depressed (C)."

"My children won't follow my suggestions (A) and make me very angry (C)."

"This traffic jam (A) really frustrates me (C)."

Ellis suggests that the key to stress is our irrational *Beliefs*, or as we say, our distorted thoughts and cognitions. Ellis's A-B-C account of stress might look like this:

"My boss rejected my report. (A) I think I should always be complimented for my efforts, even when I make a few mistakes. (B) I got depressed when my expectations were not met. (C)"

"My children won't follow my suggestions. (A) I think children should always obey their parents. (B) I got very angry. (C)"

"I was stuck in a traffic jam. (A) I think everyone else on the highway should be considerate, recognize that I'm in a hurry, and let me pass. (B) I wish I could just ram my car into them. (C)"

I find it more useful to consider a slightly different formula. Like Ellis, we begin with activating stimuli, or Cues. Cues can be either early warning signs that a stressful event or situation is down the road, near, although not actually present, or signals that a stressor is just about to occur. As for Ellis, a cue can be a external activating event such as a fire alarm, a letter of warning from the bank, or a bad grade on a quiz. But cues can also be feelings/symptoms, thoughts, and behaviors.

When stress comes, we respond. Our responses consist primarily of what we think and do, our thoughts and behaviors.

Our responses have consequences, that is, costs and benefits. Like cues, consequences can be aspects of the external situation (losing the job, failing the test, etc.) as well as feelings/symptoms, thoughts, and behaviors.

Here are some examples of our Cue–Response–Consequence formula:

"Whenever I get that tinge of fear in my stomach at work [FEELING/SYMPTOM CUE], I know this means my boss is going to criticize me."

"My boss yells at me and I freeze up. I just don't know what to say, and I leave the room [BEHAVIOR RESPONSE]."

"After this entire frustrating encounter is over, I start thinking about how stupid my behavior was. I start putting myself down [THOUGHT CONSEQUENCE]."

"Whenever I start thinking how I don't have what it takes [THOUGHT CUE], I know it's going to be a rough day at school."

"I take extra time getting to school, avoiding actually going to class. I arrive at class 15 minutes late. I start thinking that the professor is going to be extremely critical of me and everyone is going to think I'm stupid [BEHAVIOR AND THOUGHT RESPONSE]."

"I start sweating and getting really anxious. I get really nervous. [FEELING/SYMPTOM CONSEQUENCE]."

Once again, we will use this formula:

CUES - - - - - - - - - - -RESPONSE - - - - - - - - - - CONSEQUENCES

The External Situation		The External Situation
Thoughts	Thoughts	Thoughts
Behaviors	Behaviors	Behaviors
Feelings/Symptoms		Feelings/Symptoms

It might be easier to remember that cues and consequences can be just about anything that comes before or after what one does. And a response is what one actually thinks and does in an attempt to cope.

In this chapter we focus on cognitions. Ellis (1962) and Beck (1976) propose that stress is enhanced by thinking that is irrational or unproductive or maladaptive, that is, thinking that does not effectively contribute to problem-solving. I prefer the terms "unrealistic" or "distorted."

SECTION 2: CATCHING THOUGHTS

Thoughts are often very subtle and fleeting, passing so quickly and quietly we simple fail to notice or remember them. To illustrate this point, a clinician might ask a client to describe what they were thinking just one hour ago or ask if they ever felt distressed (experiencing a backache, anxiety, depression, or irritation) without exactly knowing why. However, one thinks most of the time. Ellis (1962) and Beck (1976) describe this internal dialog as *self-talk* and *automatic thinking*. Rarely does one think a complete, fully formed sentence (let alone a paragraph) about a stressful situation. Automatic thoughts are most often fleeting fragments of more complete ideas. For example, rarely would one think a complete thought like the following:

> Yesterday my boss pulled me into his office and gave me a 15-minute lecture on how I was late every day this week. He said this was not acceptable, and as a result he fired me. I was confused about why he did this without talking with me earlier. I don't know what to do.

More likely, one's thoughts might look like this:

> Yesterday I got fired. I'm messed up.

A variety of exercises can help people "slow down" and "catch" their stressful thinking. I have listed eight roughly according to their effortfulness. It can be useful to begin with the first, and proceed to those that follow.

Cartoon Captioning

How do cartoonists communicate what their characters are thinking? By thought balloons over their heads. Beck suggests that one can draw a stick figure of oneself in a stressful situation, with a thought balloon over the head. Then, one actually writes in the balloon the thoughts that occurred. If necessary, introduce "speech boxes" to emphasize the distinction between thoughts and speech.

Cartoon captioning can be one of the easiest thought catching techniques to apply. People generally find it interesting and fun. In addition, presenting weighty stress situations in cartoon format often introduces a healthy element of objectivity and humor.

Story-Telling

A good story includes all the details, what the characters do, feel, say, and think. A clinician might illustrate this to a client with a good story recently read or seen in a movie. One describes all the details and then presents the client stress situation or event "as a good story." Humor might be introduced by suggesting that this stress story is under consideration for a major motion picture, or perhaps a soap opera. All the details are included that are necessary for actors to act out the story, including actions, feelings, speech, and thoughts of the major characters.

Fantasy Video Recorder Slowdown

A client might be asked to imagine that a video recording has been made of their thoughts, feelings, actions, and speech during a stress situation. Often when we slow a recording down, we notice details we missed. Police often use this technique to catch important details. In this exercise, one fantasizes the stress situation, deliberately slowing each step of the fantasy down. Specifically, the situation is narrated out loud in the presence of the clinician. Both clinician and client take care to keep the pace of the narration as slow as possible. When a client speeds past a part, the clinician slows it down:

CLIENT: "After my boss said 'no' to my request for a raise, I just stormed out of the office."

CLINICIAN: "Whoa, let's take that real slowly. You stormed out of the office while thinking . . ."

CLIENT: "Yes, I closed my eyes real tight, thought 'that boss is such a stupid, arrogant, and hateful individual,' made a tight fist, and slowly walked out of the door, slamming it real hard."

"Mirroring"

A client presents a stress situation or event in the third person as if it really happened to someone else. It's as if the client were looking in a mirror and objectively describing the person he or she sees as a different person, including actions, thoughts, and feelings.

Thinking Out Loud

Here the client acts out a stress encounter. Another person, such as a teammate or clinician, plays the part of any other important character. However, in addition to role-playing actions and speech, the actor also notes what he or she is thinking and feeling.

Reverse Role-Playing

A client selects another person to act out a stress event, playing his or her part. The client instructs the actor what to say and do at every step. During the role-playing exercise, he or she also describes what the actor is thinking and feeling.

Group Brainstorming

Using brainstorming principles (see previous chapter), one generates ideas as to what one might be experiencing in a stressful situation or event.

Thought Diary

One completes a daily stress diary, recording thoughts and feelings that occur for at least one stress event every day.

SECTION 3: REALITY CHECKING

Once one has identified distorted thinking, the next step is to check how realistic it is, challenge it with alternatives, and select a preferred, less stressful line of thinking. This entire process is called *cognitive change* (or "cognitive restructuring"). In Section 3 we define reality checking, both of perceived facts ("Is this *really* true?") and judgmental evaluations ("Is this *really* as bad as I thought?"). In Section 4 we consider a questionnaire that can be useful for reality checking. Section 5 reviews the complete cognitive change process.

Reality Check of Factual Conclusions

The facts of stress include the specifics of a situation and event as well as immediate causes and consequences. Such factual information also includes agency and responsibility, who did what and what happened. In realistically checking these elements, one considers resources, abilities, needs, constraints, and other facts of a situation. Finally, one realistically checks longer-term conclusions, distinguishing probabilities from speculations, guesses, assumptions, preferences, and wishes. We can see an application of reality checking of such facts in the text that follows:

Probably realistic. "Yesterday I lost my job. What a disappointment! It will take some time and effort to search the papers and find new job possibilities."

Probably unrealistic. "Yesterday I lost my job. I'll never get a job again." (How can he say he will never find a job when he hasn't started looking?)

Reality Check of Evaluations of Undesirability

Conclusions about the facts of a stressful situation (accurate or not) can be judged as good or bad, personally or morally desirable or undesirable. Such evaluations can be realistic simple preferences, or unrealistic, misplaced, and exaggerated absolutes. We can see the distinction here:

Probably realistic. "Yesterday I lost my job. What a disappointment! I have a hunch my wife will also be disappointed."

Probably unrealistic. "Yesterday I lost my job. I am a worthless person. I have failed as a husband and father." (Losing a job doesn't affect one's worth as a human being, husband, or father.)

"Must," "ought," and "should" are very tricky words because they often have hidden meaning. For example, at one level the statement "I absolutely must have a girlfriend" reflects a preference, "I desire a girlfriend." The words "absolutely must" add something to this desire, an unstated ominous "or else"—an unstated moral obligation with implied exaggerated consequence. If one were to fully clarify the statement "I absolutely must have a girlfriend" we would see that actually means "I absolutely must have a girlfriend *or else* I will live a totally lonely and unhappy life." Similarly, the statement "I should always be friendly to others" might be deciphered to mean "I should always be friendly to others . . . or else I will be morally deficient in the eyes of God (or hated by everyone, or will actually hurt others, etc.).

SECTION 4: COGNITIVE DISTORTIONS AND THE SMITH IRRATIONAL BELIEFS INVENTORY

Checking the reality of appraised facts and evaluations can be challenging. Cognitive behavior therapists, generally starting with Ellis (Ellis & Dryden, 1977), have made the task easier by listing examples of cognitive distortions (irrational beliefs). Taken together, a daunting catalog of more than 50 distortions has been named (Beck, 1973; Burns, 1990; Ellis, 1985; Ellis & Dryden, 1997; Gardner, 1957; Leahy & Holland, 2000; McMullin, 2000). I propose a general three-part model that incorporates most.

The model begins with *unrealistic desires and expections*. We may want too much or expect the unreasonable. When these wants and expectations are not met, we may display an *exaggerated negative reaction*. This in turn may be accompanied by a general sense of *fatalism and helplessness*. Here is my model, with specific component distorted thoughts in italics (See Smith Irrational Beliefs Inventory, Table 6.1).

A Three-Part Model of Distorted Thoughts

Unrealistic Desires or Expectations

We start with one's desires or expectations of what the world should be like. Two frequently mentioned distorted thoughts are Perfectionism and Childlike Fantasy. The *Perfectionist* believes things should be just so. One should not make mistakes, or should always try to meet a very high, perhaps unrealistic standard. Here is how one might challenge perfectionistic thinking.

> REALITY CHECK OF FACTUAL CONCLUSION. Who has ever reached the goal you seek? Given your resources and time, is it realistic to expect you can achieve this goal?
> REALITY CHECK OF EVALUATION. Why is it so important that this goal be achieved precisely as you desire? Are there some goals that are more important than others?

A slightly different distorted thought is *Childlike Fantasy*, the immature expectation that everything should go one's way, that everyone should be nice and love each other, and that all problems should have happy endings. All such beliefs involve thinking in terms of unrealistic *Musts, Oughts, and Shoulds*, rather than simple preferences.

> REALITY CHECK OF FACTUAL CONCLUSION. In reality, the world isn't perfect, ideal, or all-loving; things do not work this way.
> REALITY CHECK OF EVALUATION: Is it an absolutely necessity to get what you want? A more realistic evaluation might be to think of it as generally desirable to achieve one's realistic desires.

Exaggerated Negative Reaction

The two most frequently cited types of exaggerated reaction are Catastrophizing and Fortune-telling. A *Catastrophizer* unrealistically concludes that something very bad has happened; a *Fortune-teller* expects it will happen. Both turn simple frustrations into absolute disasters, sometimes aggravating distress by assuming excessive *Self-blame*. Both tend to think that *Possibilities = Probabilities* (if something bad can happen, it will, or has), obsess over possible consequences (*"What if? What if? What if?"*), or put a *Negative Spin* on even neutral or potentially positive events.

TABLE 6.1　The Smith Irrational Beliefs Inventory (SIBI)

Nearly everyone experiences stress one time or another. Think of sometime over the past two weeks when you experienced a specific stressful situation or event (not "I'm always stressed out"). What were you doing? Where were you? Who was there? What did you want? What went wrong? In the box below, NAME THE STRESSFUL SITUATION OR EVENT you have in mind.

MY STRESSFUL SITUATION OR EVENT

Often our thoughts make stress worse. Below are some common types of unproductive and distorted stress-producing thinking. Please check how much you thought each in your stress situation (in the box). Use this key:

IN MY BOXED STRESS SITUATION OR EVENT . . .

① = I DIDN'T think this way at all
② = I thought this way A LITTLE
③ = I thought this way SOMEWHAT
④ = I thought this way A LOT.

---

① ② ③ ④　1.　CHILDLIKE FANTASY: Assuming (as children may do) that everything should go your way. "Everyone should be nice and love each other." "Problems should have happy endings."

① ② ③ ④　2.　DEEP MISTRUST: Expecting that others willfully mistreat, dislike, manipulate, or take advantage of you. "Others are just out to get me." "You can't trust anyone."

① ② ③ ④　3.　NEGATIVE FORTUNE-TELLING: Consistently predicting the future negatively, typically thinking that things will never change or only get worse. "I'll fail that exam or won't get the job." "I will never be really contented."

TABLE 6.1   The Smith Irrational Beliefs Inventory (SIBI) *(Continued)*

① ② ③ ④   4. NEEDLESS PERFECTIONISM: Picking an unfairly high standard you are responsible for, even though practically no one has ever been able to achieve it. "I should never do dumb things." "It's all my responsibility and I shouldn't be making mistakes."

① ② ③ ④   5. HELPLESSNESS: Believing you just can't cope by yourself and need much help and support from others. "I can't deal with things by myself." "My situation is so bad that I need someone else to take over and solve my problems for me." "I just can't cope."

① ② ③ ④   6. IMPERFECTIONS / FEELINGS = UNLOVABILITY. Feeling that you are basically defective and flawed. Believing you have strong or unusual negative or positive feelings that make you unlovable to others if they find out."If people knew what I am really like, they would never like me." "I keep my strong or unusual feelings to myself, otherwise people may not like or accept me."

① ② ③ ④   7. CATASTROPHIZING. Turning simple frustrations, irritations, and disappointments into unbearable disasters and catastrophes. "I didn't get that raise (good grade, date, etc.); therefore it is the end of the world for me." "Things didn't turn out like I wanted; this is a disaster."

① ② ③ ④   8. SPECIAL PRIVILEGE. Feeling like you have a special privilege or entitlement or that you always deserve more respect or attention than you get. "Everyone should always treat me nicely." "I should get what I want in life."

① ② ③ ④   9. TASK EXAGGERATION: Treating simple barriers or challenges as overwhelming or insurmountable. "I don't break a problem down into manageable parts. I see the whole thing as overwhelming." "If I can't immediately solve it all, why try?"

① ② ③ ④   10. UNREALISTIC ISOLATION. Feeling that you are different and isolated from the rest of the world. You cannot have lovers, friends, or satisfying relationships. "I just don't belong." "I'm different from others."

① ② ③ ④   11. POSSIBILITIES = PROBABILITIES. Thinking that if it is possible for something to go wrong, then it is probable. "If I can mess up, I will." "If there's any chance things won't go my way, they won't." "I can never zcope. That I got through my most recent crisis is an exception that doesn't count."

① ② ③ ④   12. "MUSTS, OUGHTS, AND SHOULDS": Turning simple honest desires, wants, and expectations into absolute musts, oughts, and shoulds. "I must be successful (or famous, rich, powerful, religious, loved, healthy, etc.)." vs. "It sure would be nice to be successful (famous, rich, etc.), but that may or may not happen." Or: "I should be more likable (hard-working, tidy, responsible, family-oriented, etc.) vs. "I would like to be more likable (etc.)

TABLE 6.1 *(Continued)*

① ② ③ ④   13. RIGID, EITHER / OR THINKING: Viewing events or people in all-or-nothing right-or-wrong terms and not considering"shades of gray." "Unless I can fix myself or my situation completely, I won't even try." "It feels like absolutely nobody can ever be trusted."

① ② ③ ④   14. NEEDLESS OTHER-BLAMING: Looking for someone else to blame when things don't go right. "My husband is to blame for the way I feel now," or "My mother caused all my problems."

① ② ③ ④   15. UNREALISTIC NEED FOR LOVE AND APPROVAL. Having a need for love and approval that is so strong that it influences much of your day and what you say and do with others. "I must have the love and approval of others." "I think I should always try to get people to love or accept me. "

① ② ③ ④   16. NEGATIVE SPIN. Arbitrarily and pessimistically putting a negative interpretation on events, even though they may be neutral or positive. "This is not turning out the way I want." "I always look at the dark side of things."

① ② ③ ④   17 EMOTION-DISTORTED THINKING: Letting your negative feelings color and distort how you see the facts. "I feel so depressed that everything I do seems inadequate." "Sometimes my needs and emotions take over and I just don't see myself or others objectively."

① ② ③ ④   18. IGNORING CONTRARY EVIDENCE: Focusing on negative evidence while ignoring or discounting equally relevant positive evidence. "No one likes me. The fact that you like me doesn't count." "I'll never succeed. My college degree and job aren't important ."

① ② ③ ④   19 NEEDLESS SELF-BLAME: Making a problem worse by needlessly blaming yourself for negative events, shortcomings, or imperfections; failing to see that some events have other, complex causes. "It's bad enough that my marriage ended, it's even worse that it's all my fault." "Sure things are bad. They are even worse because I feel that I'm totally responsible."

① ② ③ ④   20. REGRETTING THE PAST Focusing on past problems rather than what you have or can do now. Believing there is little you can do to improve the future given the powerful impact of past misfortunes. "So many things have gone wrong that there's not much I can do now to cope." or "My life has been filled with frustration and difficulties, and there is little I can do about it. "

① ② ③ ④   21. MINIMIZING/AVOIDING: Understating or avoiding the true significance of events resulting in problems eventually becoming worse through inaction. "That problem's just in my mind." "I'll get over it." "Things will get better on their own."

TABLE 6.1   The Smith Irrational Beliefs Inventory (SIBI) *(Continued)*

① ② ③ ④   22. MIND-READING: Believing you know what others want, think, or feel without asking. "He doesn't like me. I just know it." "You're trying to analyze me. I can see it in your smile."

① ② ③ ④   23. WHAT IF? WHAT IF? WHAT IF? Constantly asking "What if?" something happens, and failing to be satisfied with any of the answers. "Yeah, but what if I get anxious?" or "What if I freeze up?"

① ② ③ ④   24. FATALISM: Believing that the uncontrollable powers of fate determine the present, and that there is little you can do about it. "No use in trying to make things better; it's been fated to happen this way." "It's my lot in life (my social background, genes, family) to have these problems, and there's not much I can do to change that."

Can you think of any additional types of unproductive or distorted stress-producing thinking? Please list them below:

REALITY CHECK OF FACTUAL CONCLUSION. How does the Fortune-teller know for sure only bad things will happen? Unexpected things happen. Why set yourself up for failure? Just because it is possible something might go wrong, doesn't mean it will.

REALITY CHECK OF EVALUATION: Is the expected outcome actually a disaster, or is it simply frustrating and less than ideal?

Fatalism and Helplessness

The third category of stress-producing negative thinking is the distorted thought that one cannot do anything about an unmet desire or expectation. The *Fatalistic* person unrealistically focuses on the uncontrollable impact external and historical forces have on one's life; the *Helpless* individual focuses on the resulting belief that one just can't cope or must be taken care of by others.

REALITY CHECK OF FACTUAL CONCLUSION. Actually, everyone can cope with something, and even successful coping with small things shows that we have the potential for coping with others. After all, Rome was not built in a day. Although an entire problem might seem overwhelming, taking it in small steps can make it manageable.

REALITY CHECK OF EVALUATION. People who feel needlessly help-less often have a low opinion of themselves and irrationally evalu-ate themselves as weak or worthless.

Direct contributors to Fatalism and Helplessness are the tendency to *Blame Others,* blame and *Regret the Past,* or engage in *Task Exaggeration.*

Distorated Isolation: A Variation of the Basic Model

Some distorted thoughts primarily involve other people. Distorted isola-tion is a cluster of interpersonal distortions that generally follow the three-part model just described. Here the initial unrealistic desire/expectation is an *Unrealistic Need for Love and Approval.* This distorted thought may eventually contribute to the exaggerated negative reaction of *Unrealistic Isolation,* the feeling that one is isolated, different, and cannot form satis-fying relationships. Finally, one may feel Fatalistic and Helpless about this situation because of a *Deep Mistrust* toward others or a belief that *Personal Imperfections or Feelings* drive others away.

REALITY CHECK OF FACTUAL CONCLUSION. What is your basic defect and flaw that keeps you alone? Is it really a defect, or is it a very human trait, something many people have?
REALITY CHECK OF EVALUATION: Are you exaggerating the seri-ousness of your perceived flaw? Might it be seen as a minor imperfection, idiosyncrasy, or even one distinctive aspect of your personality?

General Distorted Thoughts

Some distorted thoughts can fit into any of our three categories. For example, *Rigid Either/or Thinking* refers to the tendency to think in black and white terms, accepting no middle ground or ambiguity. Such think-ing can characterize Perfectionism ("It's either perfect, or not worth doing"), Catastrophizing ("It's either the end of the world or nothing"), Unrealistic Isolation ("Either people love me or hate me"), or Fatalism and Helplessness ("Either I'm in control or totally helpless."). Similarly, *Ignoring Contrary Evidence,* or the propensity to look at negative evidence only, can be a part of Perfectionism ("Only people who try to be perfect at everything actually prosper"), Fortune-telling ("Every time I go to school I make a fool of myself"), Unrealistic Isolation ("No one in the entire world finds me likable"), and Helplessness ("I have never suc-ceeded at a task I did all by myself").

The Smith Irrational Beliefs Inventory (SIBI) measures these groups of cognitive distortions. Currently there are no scoring instructions. A useful guide is to treat any score of "2" or higher as a sign that the corresponding distorted thought may need attention. See Table 6.2 for a tentative organization of distorted thoughts according to the conceptualization just presented. Appendix A summarizes one study that offers provisional support for our model of cognitive distortions.

The Vicious Circle of Cognitive Distortions

Negative thoughts breed other negative thoughts. Once one engages in distorted thinking, the door to other distorted thoughts has been opened. For example, a person might have thoughts of Unrealistic Isolation ("I am different and cannot be a part of any community.") If this were absolutely and unvariably true, one might also realistically engage in Helpless thinking ("I just can't cope with my problems. There's nothing I can do.") And if a person were in fact actually Isolated *and* Helpless, it is likely they would also engage in Fortune-telling ("No matter what I do, it will turn out bad.") Given the way distorted thoughts can be part of a vicious circle, it is important to have reality-checking skills to break the pattern.

Discovering One's Own, Unique, Distorted Thinking and Belief Patterns

Once a client has had practice identifying cognitive distortions, he or she often can think of types of distortions not listed. This is an excellent indication that the basic idea underlying cognitive distortions has been mastered, and should be encouraged. Often distortions are highly situation specific:

No one at work has the slightest awareness of my difficulties.

Everything happens too fast.

I can be easily hurt and must be treated very gently.

Distorted thoughts can also be aggravated and maintained by more general beliefs. For example, a client might uncover the following specific distorted thoughts:

"I need the approval of guys I date in order for me to accept myself."

"I need my family to accept me before I can accept myself."

"I need my boss to accept me before I can accept myself."

These might reflect a more general and encompassing distorted theme:

"I am just not lovable."

TABLE 6.2 Categories of Irrational Beliefs

The Basic Three-Part Model

Unrealistic Desires/Expectations
  Childlike fantasy (item 1)
  Needless perfectionism (4)
  Special privilege (8)
  "Musts, oughts, and should's" (12)

Exaggerated Negative Reaction
  Negative fortune-telling (3)
  Catastrophizing (7)
  Possibilities = probabilities (11)
  Negative spin (16)
  Needless self-blame (19)
  What if? What if? What if? (23)

Fatalism and Helplessness
  Helplessness (5)
  Task exaggeration (9)
  Needless other-blaming (14)
  Regretting the past (20)
  Fatalism (24)

Distorted Isolation

  Unrealistic need for love and approval (Unrealistic Desire/Expectation; 15)
  Unrealistic isolation (Exaggerated Negative Reaction; 10)
  Deep mistrust (Fatalism and Helplessness; 2)
  Imperfections or certain feelings = unlovability (Fatalism and Helplessness; 6)

General

  Rigid, either/or thinking (13)
  Emotion-distorted thinking (17)
  Ignoring contrary evidence (18)
  Minimizing/avoiding (21)
  Mind-reading (22)

Aaron Beck (1993) has termed such themes "schemas," or basic core beliefs. It can be very useful to note that some distorted thoughts can reoccur as general encompassing themes, and that these themes almost function as personal hidden philosophies of life.

Distorted, Dysfunctional, Silly, Crazy, Stupid, "Stinkin' Thinkin'"

Once clients have gained some practice in understanding and applying reality checks to stressful thinking, they can find it useful to decide what to call this overall process. Although we have used somewhat formal labels such as "irrational," "maladaptive," and "distorted," clients usually prefer their own terms, often quite personal, colorful, and tinged with emotion. Ideally, one picks a title that is somehow linked with basic beliefs, whether they be philosophical or religious. Here are some examples of labels one might consider:

"Mistaken thinking."

"This kind of thinking is just crazy thinking."

"It's just stupid to think this way."

"These kinds of thoughts are simply silly."

"This is just being childish."

"Sinful thinking. To think this way is a 'sin,' it goes against God's will to see the world as it really is, and to live our full potential."

"This thinking is just out of touch, living in fantasy land."

"Dishonest thinking."

"Unhealthy thinking. These kinds of thoughts contribute to stress, which contributes to illness."

"Unloving thinking. Distorted thinking gets in the way of loving, caring, long-lasting relationships."

"Unproductive thinking. Such thinking is just a waste of time and doesn't do anything to contribute to a solution."

"This is weak thinking. Power thinking meets the reality check."

"This is 'stinkin' thinkin.'"

There is a value in coming up with one's own, personalized label for thinking that fails reality checks. Personalized labels individualize the process of identifying and challenging stressful thoughts. Reality checking becomes more personally meaningful and salient. A client is more likely to counter stressful thoughts highly and fully motivated, rather than as an abstract academic exercise. Of course, one should not engage in a form of distorted evaluation when creating a name for one's distorted thinking. Always remember that a distorted thought is not the end of the world, a personal imperfection, a flaw that chases others away, and so on (that's "stinkin' thinkin'!). The labels we have considered can be useful when applied with a certain sense of humor.

SECTION 5: CHECK–CHALLENGE–SELECT: CHANGING DISTORTED THINKING

Cognitive therapists have invented hundreds of strategies for helping others change distorted unrealistic thoughts (Leahy & Holland, 2000;

McMullin, 2000). Stressful thinking can be a deeply entrenched habit that requires much practice to counter. It is likely that success at changing such habits is enhanced when one frequently practices many strategies. In previous sections we introduced the idea of checkingthe reality of facts and evaluations. Here we consider the entire process of cognitive change, which can be summarized:

CHECK—CHALLENGE—SELECT

When helping others with their own distorted and unrealistic thinking, I recommend not providing direct judgements ("Your thinking is distorted and does not take into account the evidence.") Instead, the clinician helps the client develop the skills of evaluating their own thinking. We now consider each step, using nontechnical language appropriate for clinical application.

STEP 1: Check

The first step involves simply focusing on the degree to which factual conclusions and evaluations are rational and adaptive, that is, realistic. I strongly recommend attacking a problem thought from many angles. This requires not only considerable practice in applying a technique, but skill at switching from one technique to another. In sum, the goal here is to reach the conclusion that "this thought is unrealistic."

Clearly Define and Appropriately Differentiate Facts and Evaluations

OBJECTIVELY AND CONCRETELY DEFINE TERMS THAT ARE VAGUE, GLOBAL, AND JUDGMENTAL

"I am a complete failure." Just what is a complete failure? "I got an F on my first exam." "She is evil." Define evil. "She didn't return my phone call."

EVALUATE BEHAVIORS, NOT PERSONS

"I failed as a person." vs. "I failed the midterm." "I am a terrible husband." vs. "I made a mistake with my wife."

DISTINGUISH FACTS FROM EVALUATIONS

"Not getting that loan makes my life unbearable." vs. "Not getting that loan means I can't buy that car this year."

DISTINGUISH GLOBAL EVALUATIONS FROM SIMPLE PREFERENCES

"It is the end of the world for me because I did not have a date last night." vs. "I am frustrated because I did not have a date last night."

EXAMINE CONTRADICTIONS BETWEEN THOUGHTS

"I want to be perfect in everything and never give up a task." Trying to be perfect at many tasks means you will have to be less than perfect at others (in order to have enough time to be perfect).

Gather Evidence, Explore Presumed Causal Links and Logical Ramifications

DEFINE ACCEPTABLE EVIDENCE

"People think I am a dork." Let's define our terms; what's a dork? "People think that I don't know what I am talking about when I'm having a discussion." What things would people say or do to prove to you and others that they think this way?

WEIGH EVIDENCE FOR AND AGAINST A THOUGHT

"People think that I don't know what I am talking about when I'm having a discussion." Let's list all the times this week you had clear evidence that people thought you did not know what you were talking about, and all the times when people thought you did know what you were talking about. "This week no one said I was stupid, walked away, or told others I didn't know things. Evidence against: people talked with me, and asked me questions implying that I must know something. This happened about five or six times this week."

APPLY SAME STANDARD TO EVERYONE ELSE

"I am a weak person because I can't immediately calm down whenever I'm in a stressful situation." Is it reasonable to call everyone weak when they can't immediately calm down in stressful situations? Why or why not? "I do not have a wife; therefore I must be unlovable." Is everyone who does not have a wife unlovable?

DISTINGUISH PROBABILITIES FROM POSSIBILITIES

"I will get nervous during the interview and forget everything." vs. "I will probably get a bit nervous during the interview, but it is very unlikely I will forget everything."

CONSIDER FULL CHAIN OF CONSEQUENCES, AND EVALUATE

"I didn't get the raise, and that's the end of the world." What's the consequence of not getting the raise? "I won't be able to fix the car or remodel the basement." What's the consequence of that? "My car will be less comfortable and more noisy when I drive. I won't be able to watch TV in the basement with my friends." What's the consequence, is that so bad? "I'll still get places in my car, I'll still be able to entertain."

TEST THE THOUGHT WITH AN EXPERIMENT

"When I talk to my friends, they really don't want to talk with me and want to be somewhere else." Let's design an experiment to test this out. "The next 10 friends and acquaintances I start to talk to, I could suggest, 'I know you might be a bit busy, would you rather continue this later sometime?' I could record each time the other person agrees and walks away."

EXAMINE IF PAST WORRIES OR PREDICTIONS HAVEN'T COME TRUE OR ARE NO LONGER IMPORTANT

"I know I'll mess up this date. I'm always worrying about how things will go wrong." Let's look at past things you have or might have worried about. Let's see which have actually come true. Which are no longer important to you?

HOW WOULD OTHERS EVALUATE THE QUALITY OF ONE'S EVIDENCE AND THINKING?

"I'm just no good at work." Why is that? "Well, yesterday I was five minutes late, last week I couldn't find a report I'm working on, and today I forgot to make a phone call." Imagine you are (name a friend you can trust). Realistically, how would this person rate you if they knew these facts about your work?

SURVEY OTHERS' OPINIONS

"My chances of getting a job are ruined now that I got a C in my accounting class." Let's check this out with some other people. Who are some people you could ask if this is true? "My current boss, my instructor, classmates, friends who have graduated."

Explore Underlying Core Beliefs or Schemas
THE "WHY" QUESTION

If we were to examine a catalog of someone's distorted thoughts, patterns would emerge. People often have certain types of thoughts. This can indicate the presence of underlying distorted core beliefs (or "schema"). Identifying a core distorted belief can speed the process of considering the reality of facts and evaluations. One simply notes a negative thought, and then attempts to answer this question: "Why is this important to me?" Whatever answer emerges, ask again, "Why is this important to me?" When asked repeatedly, the "Why question" at first unearths similar parallel concerns and then a core belief. For example:

"Joan criticized me at work and I got upset." Why is that important to you? "Because I don't want Joan to criticize me at work, and I don't want to get upset." Why is that important to you? Why don't you want Joan to criticize you at work? "Actually, I don't want anyone at work to criticize me." Why is it important to you that people at work don't criticize you? "It is important to me that I be liked by everyone. I need to be liked."

Once one has identified what appears to be a more general or abstract core belief ("I need to be liked"), the inquiry is stopped. Then one can consider how realistic this core belief actually is.

THE "SO WHAT" QUESTION

A very similar way of pursuing underlying core beliefs is to repeatedly ask "If this were true (or were to really happen), so what? What would be so bad about that? And, what would be so bad about that? And that?" Returning to the previous example:

"Joan criticized me at work and I got upset." What is so bad about that? "When Joan criticizes me, she is disapproving of my work." What's so bad about that? "When Joan criticizes my work, I feel like she is disapproving of me." What's so bad about that? "I want other people to like and approve of me."

Again, one stops asking the question when an encompassing abstract core belief has been uncovered.

STEP 2: Challenge

Once a client has uncovered weaknesses in a negative thought, it is appropriate to move ahead and consider alternatives. Here the goal is not to select one replacement thought, but continue the process of attacking a negative thought. However, the strategy shifts from finding flaws in a client's thinking to challenging it with more realistic and adaptive alternative ways of thinking. Put simply, one explores options that would enable one to conclude "there are more realistic ways of thinking about this."

Generate Neutral or Positive Alternatives that Counter Negative Thought

BRAINSTORM OTHER SOURCES OF RESPONSIBILITY, CONTRIBUTING CAUSES, MITIGATING FACTORS, CONSEQUENCES, OR REASONABLE WAYS OF EVALUATING THE SITUATION

"My child got a poor grade in reading. I'm a failure as a parent." Let's think of other factors that might have contributed to your child's bad grade. "The friends she hangs around with . . . having too many extracurricular activities . . . not scheduling enough reading homework . . . needing glasses . . . having a teacher she doesn't like."

ANTICIPATE REALISTIC POSSIBLE FUTURES THAT PUT THINGS IN PERSPECTIVE

"Yes, we've talked about this for quite some time. My employer is going out of business and I won't have a job next month." I know this is a great concern for you, but let's stand back and think about a year, two years, even five years from now. What kinds of things might happen that would cause you to look back at today and say "that wasn't so bad after all"? "I hope I'll be married with some children. I certainly will have another job, hopefully one that is stable."

CONSIDER WHAT GOOD REMAINS (OR WHAT IS STILL POSSIBLE) EVEN IF THE WORST HAPPENS?

"I get my performance review tomorrow. I know I've made a few mistakes, so I don't expect a glowing review." So, what's the worst thing that could happen? "I could get a bad review and be asked to leave the program." Even if that happens, is there anything positive for you left? "Yes, I still have my family and friends. I know how to look for work elsewhere."

EXAMINE WHAT MIGHT BE WORSE

"I was turned down for that promotion yesterday." I understand how that might be frustrating, but it's not the worst thing that could happen. "Yes, I could have been fired, demoted, transferred out of state, put in a smaller office, or given a bad review."

COMPARE WITH OTHERS WHO MIGHT BE WORSE OFF

"I had a fender bender with my new car yesterday. I felt awful." Well, think of all the other people in your situation who might be worse off. "People have far more serious accidents, no insurance, no alternative transportation."

CONSIDER WHAT IS POSSIBLY FUNNY ABOUT THIS SITUATION

"I was in the grocery store with a cart full of canned goods. As I turned the corner, I bumped into another cart. My cart turned over, spilling everything. I felt so embarrassed and stupid." Let's look at this from a different perspective. How could have this been funny? "I could have accused the other cart of not using proper traffic signals, causing an accident."

Consider Adaptive Value

ASK HOW DOES IT HELP YOU BY FOCUSING ON YOURSELF AS CAUSE?

Even if you believe you are responsible for this situation, how does it contribute to helping you come up with some sort of solution? How does it help you cope with other problems, or generally make things better?

ASK HOW DOES IT HELP YOU BY FOCUSING ON THESE CONSEQUENCES?

Even if you believe the consequences you fear, how does this belief contribute to helping you come up with some sort of solution? How does it help you cope with other problems, or generally make things better?

HOW DOES THINKING THIS WAY CONTRIBUTE TO IMPROVED SELF-ESTEEM?

Even if this situation were true, does thinking this way needlessly hurt your self-esteem? Is there another way of thinking that may not hurt your opinion of yourself?

Accept Situation

ACCEPT THINGS THAT CANNOT CHANGE

Perhaps there are some things you cannot change.

CONSIDER THE BENEFITS OF ACCEPTING THINGS FOR NOW

Perhaps it is best to accept some problems as they are for the time being, take something of a break, and deal with them at a better time later.

CONSIDER THE BENEFITS OF NOT TRYING TO CHANGE A STRESSFUL SITUATION NOW

Perhaps trying to deal with the entire stressful situation now is not the best strategy.

CONSIDER THE ADVANTAGES OF AN INCREMENTAL APPROACH

Let's consider this problem in realistic steps, and change what can be changed now.

When Negative Thinking Persists: Role-Play Checks and Challenges

The preceding techniques of reality checking and challenging are relatively direct, and often are sufficient to evoke productive consideration of realistic and productive alternative thoughts. However, some individuals persist with negative thinking, even after sincere checks and challenges. This is most likely to occur when such help is presented as directive advice rather than as an invitation to engage in a mutual experiment. When a client continues to engage in distorted thinking, it can be helpful to engage in role-play acting. This act requires breaking out of the role of "complainer" or "nay-sayer," and tentatively taking on a potentially more productive role. Here are three role-playing strategies:

CONDUCT A LAWYER'S DEFENSE

Imagine you have been hired as an attorney to defend yourself. What is the strongest case you can make even if you aren't entirely convinced of it?

DO A DOUBLE ROLE PLAY

I (counselor/trainer) will play your role, and you take the role of an objective friend (name person). I will then argue in favor of your line of thinking, and you present the contrary position, challenging what I say.

ROLE PLAY A SITUATION AS IF STRESSFUL THOUGHT WERE NOT AS SERIOUS AS ONCE THOUGHT

Let's act out your stressful situation, you playing the role of yourself. Only let's change one thing. Pretend that you actually do not believe the stressful distorted line of thinking we have been considering.

STEP 3: Select

Once one has disputed a negative thought, and considered a full range of more realistic alternatives, the next step is to pick a realistic replacement thought. This thought should feel right to the individual, which is likely if one has engaged in the effort of working through all the preceding steps. Selecting a replacement thought does not automatically mean that one will no longer entertain the negative thought. One must practice, a topic we consider in the next section.

When to Switch to Problem-Solving, Relaxation, or Worry-Stopping

A client who attempts to check or challenge distorted thinking may quickly find that their thinking turns into an attempt to define a problem. When this happens, it can be unproductive to continue the task of checking and challenging thoughts; instead, one might start the process of problem-solving (taking a problem-solving orientation; defining a problem, brainstorming, selecting a solution; chapter 5).

Alternatively, efforts at checking and challenging distorted thinking can heighten somatic and cognitive arousal, which in itself can contribute to further negative rumination. At this point, it can be useful to simply cease and pursue relaxation training (chapter 4). Another option might be to deploy worry-stopping techniques considered in SECTION 7 of this chapter.

SECTION 6: COGNITIVE APPROACHES AND CUE–RESPONSE–CONSEQUENCES

Armed with cognitive stress management tools, we can now consider their application. I recommend applying the "C–R–C" formula we use throughout this book:

Cue–Response–Consequence

The first step in application is to acquire data on existing thought patterns. For a few days, one completes a day-end diary of recalled stress events, indicating for each the Cue, Response, and Consequence. When specifying one's response, it is of particular importance to identify cognitions and behaviors, what one thought and did. Consequences are the resulting feelings, symptoms, thoughts, feelings, and situational changes that may have been brought about. Figure 6.1 (pp. 130–131) illustrates a simple form that can be used.

The next step is to consider thoughts to counter those that contributed to stress. One then completes a slightly revised diary recording thoughts and counter thoughts, as well as behaviors, feelings and symptoms, and consequences. See Figure 6.2 (pp. 132–133) for an example.

SECTION 7: STOPPING WORRY

Worry and obsessive negative thinking are typically among the first signs that one is harboring a wide variety of distorted beliefs. What can a client do when obsessive negative thinking continues, even after trying the strategies suggested in this chapter? Obsessive thinking can be seen as a bad and unwanted habit. At times worries persist because they have generalized to many cues, and other times because of rewarding consequences. Consider the minor habit of nervously scratching one's head. A person may begin scratching his or her head while driving the morning rush hour to work. This behavior is unwittingly rewarded if it distracts him or her from fear about getting into an accident, arriving late at work, and so on. Sitting in the car also becomes a reminder cue to start scratching. However, head-scratching generalizes to other cues, such as taking the bus, waiting for the bus, waiting for your boss, and so on. Eventually, head-scratching has become a continuing habit because it has generalized to many cues.

In a similar fashion, obsessive negative thinkers perhaps begin their habit in certain, restricted circumstances, for example, worrying before taking a bus. Worry was then rewarded by a variety of short-term pay-offs. It may distract one from completing an unpleasant task, divert attention from uncomfortable choices, and give the false sense of security that one is actually accomplishing something. Eventually worrying, like head-scratching, generalizes to a wide range of cues.

In this section we consider how to stop the worry response by modifying what comes before (the cue) and what comes after (the consequence).

Modifying the Cue: Worry Sessions

Thomas Borkovec (Borkovec, 1985; Borkovec, Wilkinson, Folensbee, & Lerman, 1983) has developed an exercise for limiting worry that is based on cues that can serve as worry triggers. The goal of this exercise is to limit the number of cues that trigger worry. Here are the instructions:

1. Observe your thinking throughout the day to identify worry cues.
2. Then set aside a half-hour worry period at the same time and in the same place every day. This special time is *reserved for intensive worry*.
3. Postpone worrying until the scheduled worry period.
4. Outside of the worry period, replace worrisome thoughts with focused attention on the task at hand or anything else in the immediate environment.

The goal of setting up this exercise is to isolate worrying so that it is associated with only a limited set of cues.

Modifying the Consequences: Thought Stopping

Another strategy, *thought stopping* (Cautela & Wisocki, 1977), focuses on modifying the consequences of worry. Habitual negative thinking is often maintained by short-term payoffs, for example, the false sense of security of doing something about a problem or of feeling in control. One way of stopping the chain of worry is to change the consequences from positive to negative.

In thought stopping one deliberately follows worry with a simple *aversive* consequence. It is best to do this exercise in private where others will not be disturbed. One begins by placing a bracelet-sized rubber band on a wrist. The entire procedure takes three sessions.

Session One

1. Make a list of negative thoughts that you feel are out of your control. Example:

> "I'm not going anywhere."
> "Everyone thinks I am stupid."
> "I can only blame myself."
> "This is the end of the world."

2. Then pick a target negative thought, one to eliminate. Example:

> "Everyone thinks I am stupid."

3. Consider why you want to stop this negative thought. See Sections 1–4. It is important you do a reality check and recognize how the thought is distorted. Example:

> "It is silly to believe that everyone thinks I am stupid. I am actually brighter than many, if not most, people. This type of thinking becomes a self- fulfilling prophecy. I think others believe I am stupid, so I act stupid, confirming my fears."

4. Relax and wait a few seconds. Deliberately start thinking the worry. Just when you start thinking it, yell the word STOP! as loud as you can and snap the rubber band. Yes, yell it out loud! I know this is disruptive, and even a bit amusing, but that is the point. By yelling STOP! You break the chain. Be sure to do this in private.

I have tried a somewhat more gentle version of this intervention. Instead of yelling STOP!, try laughing out loud for two full minutes (ideally with a clinician present). Such forced laughter is at first a bit awkward, but after about a minute you may begin to sense the absurdity of the exercise and laughter acquires a certain detached quality that can actually help you look at stressful problems a bit more objectively. I call my variation of the STOP! exercise the HA! exercise.

5. Sit and wait. Relax. Repeat yelling STOP! (or HA!) and snapping the rubber band if worrying starts again.

Session Two

1. Relax and let your mind wander. The moment the worry thought spontaneously emerges, again say STOP!, this time in a normal voice, and snap the rubber band.
2. When the worry thought appears again, this time yell STOP! as one did in the first session. This can be done several times.

Session Three

1. Relax and let your mind wander. Do not try to think anything. When the worry thought comes to mind, simply *think* STOP! very loudly in the mind while snapping the rubber band.
2. When the worry thought emerges again, simply think STOP! and omit the rubber band.

Preliminary Assessment Form (Description of a stress situation before cognitive stress management has been applied)

Cue	Response		Consequences
Situation, Thoughts, Behaviors, Symptoms/Feelings	Thoughts	Behaviors	Situation, Thoughts, Behaviors, Feelings/Symptoms

Practice Form (After distorted thoughts have been challenged and replaced)

Cue	Response			Consequences
Situation, Thoughts, Behaviors, Symptoms/Feelings	Thoughts	Replacement Thoughts	Behaviors	Situation, Thoughts, Behaviors, Symptoms/Feelings

FIGURE 6.1 Diary forms for cognitive stress management.

Preliminary Assessment Form

Cue	Response		Consequences
Situation, Thoughts, Behaviors, Symptoms/Feelings	Thoughts	Behaviors	Situation, Thoughts, Behaviors, Feelings/Symptoms
I walked up to the office where the interview took place.	*I thought: "I'm going to fail. The interviewer knows all my weaknesses. I have no idea what to say. I'll never get a job."*	*I entered the office very slowly, looking at my feet, avoiding eye-to-eye contact.*	*I felt panic. It felt like the end of the world. My stomach was upset. I completed the interview. I was preoccupied with worry about my weaknesses. I could have looked directly at the interviewer and asked him some questions that illustrated I understood the job requirements. Why didn't I do that? Stupid! I walked home and avoided my wife.*

Practice Form

Cue	Response		Behaviors	Consequences
Situation, Thoughts, Behaviors, Symptoms/Feelings	Thoughts	Replacement Thoughts	Behaviors	Situation, Thoughts, Behaviors, Symptoms/Feelings
I walked up to the office where the interview took place	I thought "I'm going to fail. The interviewer knows all my weaknesses. I have no idea what to say. I'll never get a job."	Then, I counted with these thoughts: "STOP! The worst that can happen is that I might stumble on a few answers. Even than it will be a good learning experience. I have a question sheet with me I can use if I forget something. Everyone was to start learning somewhere."	I entered the office, and (as I planned) walked deliberately to the interviewer. I made a point of looking straight at the interviewer. I Made sure I had my list of questions in hand.	There, let's review how I did. I felt nervous, but did not panic. I know I was more or less in control. I did not have a stomach ache. I remembered to look at my question sheet and ask my questions. Good! I remembered to look at the interviewer rather than at my feet. That was good. The interview went better than previous ones. I'm learning from my mistakes. I walked home and told my wife about how well I did.

FIGURE 6.2 Example of practice diary for cognitive stress management.

EXERCISES

1. Fill out a daily thought diary and do a reality check of stressful thoughts. Select replacement thoughts.

2. Try cartoon captioning and story telling (write a script) as a way of catching stressful thoughts.

3. In a group, try mirroring, thinking out loud, reverse role-playing, and group brainstorming as thought catching exercises.

4. Select 10 thoughts generated in any of the above exercises. Do a reality check on each, describing what factual conclusions and what evaluations may be unrealistic.

5. Select 10 thoughts in any of the above exercises. Identify which type of stressful thinking each illustrates. Thoughts may reflect more than one type of stressful thinking.

6. What general label do you prefer for "distorted thinking"? Why?

7. Write a script in which you check or challenge each of the 10 stressful thoughts you have listed.

8. For each stressful thought listed above, select one best replacement thought that is realistic.

9. Ask someone to describe how they deal with stress in their lives. Which of the techniques (if any) described in this chapter are illustrated?

10. In what ways can reality-checking be a centered activity, involving letting go and simple, sustained focus? Include the role of R-States.

11. In a group, divide individuals into teams of three to four individuals each. Each team first generates a problem and associated distorted thinking. Next, one team presents the problem (as a team playing the role of client or helpee) and distorted thinking. The other team plays the role of counselor or helper and attempts to check or challenge the distorted thinking involved, using the techniques presented in this chapter. Then discuss what techniques were deployed. Repeat by reversing roles.

12. Find someone to interview. Ask them to describe a recent stressful event. Using the techniques of this chapter, encourage them to describe their thoughts. Identify (not to them, but on paper) distorted thinking.

7

Review and Rehearsal

Few new skills can be directly applied to challenging real-life situations. First we need to review or rehearse. One reviews by reexperiencing a past stressor and rehearses by practicing for a future encounter. A person may witness a terrifying accident and be troubled by recurring memories and flashbacks. A review treatment for overcoming the persistent emotional upset might involve carefully reliving the accident in one's mind in a safe and relaxing environment until eventually one can calmly think about the disturbing event. Rehearsal is different. A beginning driver might deploy a rehearsal technique to overcome fear of driving. The first task is to learn to operate automobile controls. However, the task is not complete once the driver can turn on the ignition, operate the clutch, and apply the brakes. He or she must rehearse in a protected environment, first in a training vehicle (with the presence of a driving instructor), and then on relatively safe streets in daylight. Only after training and rehearsal can the beginning driver calmly venture out into the dangers of real-life traffic.

The very nature of stressors dictates that structured review and rehearsal are essential parts of stress management. Uncontrollability and unpredictability (as well as undesirability, magnitude, and clustering) are fundamental stimulus characteristics that increase the threat of actual-life stressors (chapter 2). These very characteristics reduce the likelihood that one will spontaneously recover from past encounters, or successfully cope with future incidents. Through review or rehearsal we re-experience a stressor and practice skills in predefined situations in which these key aversive stimulus characteristics are artificially minimized. Doing so

---

[1] Note that in some situations one may directly apply new coping strategies without prior rehearsal. For example, a student may have an unexpected job interview the next day. The day before, her dorm counselor might teach her how to relax through deep breathing, and how to think supportive, motivating, and undistorted thoughts. These skills may be applied for the first time at the interview. Such unrehearsed application is most likely to be successful for minor stressors and for individuals who have few difficulties with stress management.

enhances the likelihood of overcoming disruptive emotional upset and coping with the uncertain real world of stress. We consider three review and rehearsal strategies: exposure, desensitization, and stress inoculation.[1]

We rely on our simple C–R–C formula: Cue–Response–Consequences. To summarize, a *cue* is an early warning sign or signal to engage in some form of coping activity. For example, a student may experience considerable anxiety during an exam. An early warning sign may be the experience of cold hands, beginning worries about performance, and so on.

One's *response* consists of what we think and do to cope. Once our student notes his cold hands or performance worries, he may begin repeating realistic coping thoughts ("answer one question at a time") and take a few deep relaxing breaths.

Finally, the *consequences* of attempting to cope represent the third part of our formula. One may experience reduced anxiety, and feelings of achievement or efficacy over having completed a coping strategy, or even remembering to relax. If a coping strategy was deployed, part of the consequence can be a predetermined reinforcement. Reinforcements can range from a simple self-congratulation, to a pleasant fantasy, to a harmless pleasurable treat. Such positive consequences help counter the aversiveness of a stressor. This is the C–R–C formula:

CUES - - - - - - - - RESPONSE - - - - - - - - - - CONSEQUENCES

The External Situation		The External Situation
Thoughts	Thoughts	Thoughts
Behaviors	Behaviors	Behaviors
Feelings/symptoms		Feelings/symptoms

SECTION 1: EXPOSURE

In exposure techniques (Foa & Kozak, 1986) a client systematically reexperiences or rehearses a stressor. The initial goal is to create and sustain (without a break or relief) a relatively high level of distress throughout a session so that emotion eventually "takes its course" and dissipates. Theory predicts that if negative emotion is sustained uninterrupted for a period of time, it habituates and is eventually tuned out and is no longer noticed. One might think of the discomfort of stepping into a cold swimming pool, or from a dark room into daylight. At first the cold water, or bright sunlight, might be very uncomfortable, even shocking. However, by deliberately staying in the water or sunlight, one eventually adapts or habituates and can tolerate the stimulation. If one were to interrupt such "exposure" sessions by retreating into a warm (dark) room, the process of habituation would not work. One would feel shock and distress once again the next time one stepped into the water or sunlight. Exposure sessions work in a similar way; a client deliberately tolerates clearly timed doses of a stressor.

People often use simple versions of exposure when dealing with everyday stressors. For example, imagine a student learning to drive for the first time. She has her first session behind the wheel, with the instructor sitting in the passenger seat. Our student is a little nervous, a normal reaction in such a situation. However, at the first sign of anxiety, she does not say, "Instructor, I'm a little nervous. Let's stop the car and turn off the street so I can get out, relax, and listen to some music with a cup of tea. Then we can get in the car and continue the lesson." Instead, she puts up with the nervousness through the entire hour-long session. And her anxiety spontaneously reduces.

Here's another example in the form of an interchange between Sam and Marti. Sam is recalling a very embarrassing dinner party incident in which she spilled water on the host.

SAM: "I have to tell you about this embarrassing incident, and get it off my chest."

MARTI: "I'm all ears. Tell me what happened."

SAM: "I was at a dinner party hosted by my neighbor, Brad. There were about 10 of us sitting around the table. We were all dressed up. It was going to be such a wonderful time. The food smelled good, and several of my friends and neighbors were there. I really wanted to make a good impression, because they all knew me."

MARTI: "Sounds like a great dinner. Was the food good?"

SAM: "Please, let me stay on track. I want to get this out in the open and tell you what happened."

MARTI: "Sorry. What happened next?"

SAM: "Well, Brad, the handsome single host, asked for a glass of water. Everyone noticed he was the only one who didn't have water. So I reached over, got a glass and handed it to him. I was trying to be so helpful. It was terrible. I spilled the water. It was so awful!"

MARTI: "Did you get any water on him?"

SAM: "Yes, yes! I spilled it all over his coat. It was awful."

MARTI: "That sounds really embarrassing! I bet it was a dress coat, too."

SAM: "Oh yes, I forgot to say that. It must have been one of his best coats. Everyone sat and gasped at what happened and

Brad closed his eyes and frowned. I sat there and said nothing, and felt even more stupid for saying nothing. Eventually, Brad got up, changed coats, and came back."

MARTI: "What did he say?"

SAM: "Well, of course he said it wasn't a problem, it was just water, and the coat needed to be cleaned anyway. But the damage, the damage to me, had been done. I was mortified."

MARTI: "I can see how this could really be upsetting, with all those people watching."

SAM: "Yes, I picked up the water, and somehow it slipped out of my hand. I could hear it hit the table, and then bounce on his coat. It splashed all over!"

There are several things worth noting about this simple exposure episode. First, Sam keeps talking. She deliberately keeps her anxiety level high by giving an uninterrupted account of the incident. When Marti changes the topic by asking if the food was good, Sam quickly wants to get back to the topic. Indeed, changing the topic would have spoiled the exposure process. Remember, the key is to *maintain uninterrupted anxiety about a stress situation*. Note that at the end Sam even repeats facts she has already shared. This is also part of exposure; one sustains and repeats involvement until anxiety subsides. Also note that Marti helps the exposure process from time to time by asking for more vivid detail, and maintaining focus on the event.

Exposure applied to stress management is a bit more systematic. Generally, one creates a list or hierarchy of related situations and then relives each until tension subsides.

The Hierarchy of Situations

One first creates a hierarchy of stressful stimuli, ranked from low to high severity. The list should include about 10 or 20 items and can be ranked. The items may or may not be logically connected. For example, if one is fearful of talking to others in public, this can be used as a theme, creating the following hierarchy (rank from low to high stressfulness, 1 to 10). Here the items are not logically connected:

10. Talking to an important stranger in the presence of other strangers.
 9. Talking to an important stranger alone.
 8. Talking to an important stranger in the presence of my friends.
 7. Talking to a stranger of no particular importance, in the presence of other strangers.

6. Talking to a stranger of no particular importance in the presence of my friends.
5. Talking to a comfortable acquaintance in the presence of strangers.
4. Talking to a comfortable acquaintance in the presence of other acquaintances.
3. Talking to a friend in the presence of strangers.
2. Talking to a friend in the presence of friends.
1. Talking to a close relative.

Items can be ranked by any logical connection. In the following example, we see variations of talking with a future boss one has never met before.

10. Talking to the boss alone in the privacy of his own office.
9. Talking to the boss with my friends present.
8. Talking to the boss casually in the hallway.
7. Meeting the boss in the lounge and sharing a cup of coffee.
6. Meeting the boss on the bus.
5. Talking to the boss after having unexpectedly met him on the streets.
4. Receiving a phone call from the boss and talking to him.
3. Calling the boss on the phone.
2. Responding to an e-mail sent by the boss.
1. Receiving an e-mail from the boss.

Items can even be sequential steps in approaching a stressor. One can imagine walking to the boss's office, opening the door, shaking hands, starting small talk, engaging in serious conversation, and so on.

It can be useful to identify the variable that makes one version of a situation more threatening than another, and then use this variable as a guide for generating situations. For example, perhaps a client who is anxious about riding in an automobile identifies both the speed of travel and proximity to the driver's seat as key variables. The faster the car goes, the more anxious the client becomes. And anxiety is less when he is in the back seat, more if he in is the front passenger seat, and most if he is in the driver's seat. The identified key variable or variables can be used to create an effective hierarchy.

Next the client and clinician assemble a small stack of 10 or more sheets of paper and describe one situation on each sheet. It is important that the descriptions be concrete ("taking a seat in an airplane") rather than vague and abstract ("flying"). Descriptions should include in vivid detail the "four W's" (who, what, when, and where). Writing such situation descriptions is not unlike writing scripts for a series of episodes for a television drama. For example, in the previous example of talking to a future boss, the easiest episode might be entitled, "E-Mail from the Boss."

In its description, the client would present all the characters, what they are doing, when they are doing it, and what they are thinking and feeling. Here's an example:

E-Mail From the New Boss:
(Episode 1 of the TV Drama, "The Future Boss.")

I had just been hired for a new job as a public relations clerk in a local department store. I was to start work in a week, and was filled with apprehension and anxiety. It was a cold winter day and I was alone in the den with my computer. I turned on my computer and noticed a new e-mail. It was from my new boss. Cold beads of sweat streamed down my forehead. As I tried to open my e-mail, the computer crashed, and I had to bring my e-mail program up once again. Long minutes passed. The clock overhead was slowly ticking. I waited, not wanting to open the mail. My fingers quivered as I pressed the "open key" button. Again, long seconds ticked away as the mail opened. And finally it opened. I could see it was a detailed letter, beginning with the phrase, printed in vivid red: "Greetings to our new employee."

Descriptions should be longer than the above example and include from five to ten minutes of detail when read. Details should be relatively under control, not be subject to unexpected problems, or involve real danger to oneself and others.

Exposure Sessions

A session should last from 30 to 50 minutes. One begins the process of systematic exposure by starting with the easiest situation (the first sheet). Through imagery, a client deliberately steps into the situation, and stays with and repeats it until discomfort significantly lessens. This process is repeated on the next situation. The key is to continually expose the client to all the details of a situation without a break, like stepping into and staying in a cold swimming pool. No more than two or three situations should be included in a session. One begins the next session (no more than a week later) by starting where one left off.

How does one know when the exposure process has worked and it is time to put a situation aside and move to the next? Every 5 minutes or so the clinician asks about and notes level of discomfort (anxiety, fear, etc.) on a 10-point scale (some prefer a 100-point scale; for me, that is too many numbers). This is often called the Subjective Units of Distress Scale (SUDS). 10 is maximum discomfort, 0 is relaxation with no discomfort, and 5 is moderate discomfort. When SUDS scores have reduced by about half, it is time to do the next situation. If SUDS scores do not decline, then select an easier situation. This may involve rethinking one's hierarchy to include several less threatening items. If SUDS scores still remain high, then try desensitization (SECTION 2 in this chapter).

There are four ways of achieving exposure through imagination. This can also be done in actual life :

1. *Directed fantasy.* The clinician speaks the details out loud, presenting a sort of vivid story-telling narration, asking for additional details from time to time. Before and every 5 minutes one takes a measure of SUDS. If little anxiety is produced, details should be added to one's written description.[2]

2. *Recording.* The clinician can make an audiorecording of the session, and assign the client to play it at home two or three times a week. It should be played over and over without a break for at least 30 minutes, two or three times a week. Once again the goal is to maintain uninterrupted involvement in the situation until anxiety diminishes.

3. *Writing.* In a session a client can deliberately write about the situation, as if writing a detailed letter to a close friend. Again, all the painful details should be included. Once the "letter" is finished, put it aside and write it again. Continue this process of writing and rewriting. It is very important with this method not to "give oneself a break" and pause for rest or relief. The letter should not even include interrupting discussions of unrelated topics ("Well, the good news is that I bought a new dress yesterday"). The client is to keep the anxiety level up, without interruption.

4. *Talking.* Finally, the client can be instructed to simply talk out loud (to an imaginary person, pet, or stuffed animal) for 30–50 minutes about the stressful situation. It is important to keep talking, and keep focused on the anxiety-arousing stimuli. One might talk on a phone (unplugged). Imagine it has a poor connection, and will disconnect if it detects no speech. (Or perhaps it is some special type of phone that hangs up when it detects that the stressful situation is not being talked about.)

5. *Real-life.* Alternatively, real-life exposure involves devoting a session to actually entering the situation in actual life. If a client is afraid of public speaking, he actually gives a 30–50 minute speech. If a client is

---

[2] It is possible to increase the complexity and perceived credibility of simple exposure treatments by assigning a concurrent task that is superficially engaging and noncognitive. Others have suggested rapidly shifting one's eyes back and forth, or tapping oneself on the eyebrows, under the eyes, under the collarbone, and on the back of the hand. We have only scratched the surface of the full range of such concurrent tasks; additional possibilities include breathing alternatively through left and right nostril, standing while balancing on one foot, tapping one's foot while chewing gum, or extending one's tongue while quickly circling it in one direction then another. However, research has yet to demonstrate the superiority of any of these or other possible augmentations over simple exposure, desensitization, or stress inoculation training.

afraid of riding a car, she rides a car. This is done usually with the presence of a clinician who can check SUDS levels from time to time to determine whether extinction is taking place. Real-life exposure, like imagined exposure, first requires establishing a hierarchy of situations and proceeding from the easiest to the most challenging.

Whatever the approach, one stays in and replays a situation as long as possible until SUDS ratings have reduced by about half. It is very important that some reduction in discomfort occur, otherwise one's problem may be aggravated. The point of this approach is to learn to tolerate discomfort through prolonged and repeated exposure. Once significant reduction in discomfort has occurred for a situation, one can apply a brief reinforcement and proceed to the next situation.

As an optional addition, a client begins the session by predicting how the session will go, and ends the session with a reassessment of the prediction. This can provide an in-session opportunity to check the reality of potential distorted beliefs concerning one's performance in the targeted stressful situation.

SECTION 2: DESENSITIZATION

Desensitization (or "systematic desensitization"; Wolpe, 1959) is similar to exposure except that one begins by learning to relax deeply. It is particularly useful for situations in which initial anxiety is so high that it prevents application of a stress management technique. First the client masters relaxation and develops a mini-relaxation technique (chapter 4). Then, at the beginning of each desensitization session, he or she performs a mini-relaxation exercise in order to become relaxed again.

One begins the process of desensitization with the easiest stress situation of one's stress situation hierarchy. At the slightest cue of discomfort, one performs a mini-relaxation. When relaxed, one resumes imagined involvement. This process is repeated from session to session until one can imagine a stressor without discomfort. Some (Leahy & Holland, 2000) have suggested it is important not to do desensitization when cues for discomfort are internal (anxiety or symptoms) rather than external (approaching another person for discussion). For example, one would not use desensitization in the following public speaking situation:

Cue: Rapidly beating heart
Response: Giving a lecture and worrying about what others think
Consequence: Feeling depressed and frustrated.

However, desensitization would be appropriate in this public speaking situation:

Cue: Walking up to podium
Response: Giving a lecture and worrying about what others think
Consequence: Feeling depressed and frustrated

Again, one practices no more than 30 minutes in a session, and imagines no more than two or three situations.

SECTION 3: STRESS INOCULATION TRAINING AND RELAPSE PREVENTION

Donald Meichenbaum (1985) has developed a widely-used approach to stress management, stress inoculation training (SIT). According to Meichenbaum, stress inoculation is something like a vaccination (actually, this is also true for exposure and desensitization). An influenza vaccination consists of a small and harmless dose of an altered flu virus. The body responds to this dose by building up a resistance sufficiently strong to combat actual exposure to the flu. Similarly, in stress inoculation training, a person is exposed to a relatively innocuous version of a stressful situation and responds by building up coping skills that can then be applied to more severe stressors later on.

I like to think of stress inoculation training as a complicated version of exposure that includes relaxation (like desensitization) as well as reality-checking, coping thoughts, and a strategy we haven't considered before, relapse prevention.

Relapse Prevention

A relapse is an unexpected coping failure or setback (Marlatt & Gordon, 1984). One may "get cold feet," forget coping plans, or run into unexpected obstacles. Relapse is often a cue for negative thinking, such as:

I'll never be able to follow through on my coping plans.

This setback means I am a weak person.

I just can't cope.

The goal of relapse prevention is to use problem-solving to plan ahead for possible coping failures and setbacks. It is a strategy for helping one develop additional coping options to reduce the likelihood of giving up in the face of difficulty. In addition, a relapse strategy makes the application of stress management virtually immune to failure; even setbacks are anticipated ahead of time and considered opportunities. We consider both comeback and fallback strategies for dealing with relapse.

Comeback Strategies

A relapse becomes a cue for a special type of coping, a comeback strategy or preconsidered backup plan. For example:

> "I plan to assertively return this piece of defective merchandise tomorrow and ask for my money back. If I get cold feet and 'forget,' I will practice my relaxation exercise and try again the next day. That will give me a chance to practice my relapse prevention skills."

> "When my professor passes out the class exam, I will take three deep breaths and say to myself, 'answer the easy questions first.' If I panic and get bogged down with a hard question, I'll close my eyes, take three deep breaths, and start again. Good."

Fallback Strategies

A fallback strategy is a final relapse backup plan, one to be used even when comeback strategies do not work. We can see this in a particularly popular circus stunt:

> Imagine the tightrope walker at a circus. Although her performance might seem quite dangerous, she has a number of safety strategies. In case she slips, the balancing rod she carries can be used to latch onto the rope. She wears gloves that permit a stronger grip on the rope. If all these backups fail, there is a safety net to counter her fall. Similarly, in dealing with stress, think of a safety net strategy, what you can think and do if your backup coping strategies do not work.

Fallback strategies provide a safety net. General examples include talking to a trusted friend or relative, discussing a problem with a clinician, or writing about a problem in a personal diary. Here are some fallback thoughts (Meichenbaum, 1985; Smith, 1993a):

> Well, life goes on.
> Everyone makes mistakes.
> I still love myself (or have a loving family) in spite of my problems.
> God still loves me.
> Let's look at things in perspective. Life is too short to make too much of this problem.
> I'll treat this as water under the bridge.
> Maybe I'll learn somehow from this.

Fallback strategies help us go on living in the face of setback. They remind us not to put ourselves down for mistakes in thinking and behaving. And they prompt us to do better next time.

Stress Inoculation Training

Stress inoculation training (SIT) is like systematic exposure; however, it is a very flexible approach that incorporates relaxation, reality-checking, coping skills, and relapse prevention. Here is the version I use:

Create a Hierarchy

As in desensitization, the clinician and client construct a concrete hierarchy of increasingly stressful situations and then the client rehearses each while relaxed. Again, it is important to include all the details, like a journalist or lawyer. Think of writing a script for episodes in a TV drama, with sufficient detail that the actors and director would know what to do.

Unlike exposure or desensitization, one additionally includes appropriate statements suggesting relaxation, previously-determined reality checks for potentially distorted thinking, and coping statements. I recommend designating two to four of the situations as *relapse situations* in which the main theme is coping with relapse. For example, the following hierarchy of fear of driving includes two relapse situations:

10. Driving a car in rush hour traffic in downtown. (Most anxiety-arousing.)
9. (RELAPSE SITUATION) Driving a car in normal traffic downtown. Saying to myself, "One street at a time, I can manage this," then panicking, then taking a deep breath and repeating my fallback strategy of saying "It is normal to feel a little anxious from time to time. I can manage this."
8. Driving a car in normal traffic in a smaller town.
7. Driving a car on a busy interstate freeway.
6. (RELAPSE SITUATION) Driving a car on an interstate freeway with little traffic. I think, "Good, this is not as bad as it could be. I'm mastering my coping skills." I forget my coping skills and begin shaking at the wheel. My fallback strategy is to take a deep breath, and think, "Good. This shaking gives me a chance to practice putting my fear aside and attending to the driving task at hand."
5. Entering an empty interstate freeway from a small country road.
4. Driving down a country road with little traffic.
3. Driving out of the driveway.
2. Sitting in a car and starting the engine.
1. Walking up to a car I am about to drive. (Least anxiety-arousing.)

Meichenbaum (1985) suggests analyzing a stress situation into four phases; preparing for the stressor, confronting and handling the stressor, coping with feelings of being overwhelmed, evaluation of coping efforts and self-rewards. I have found these descriptors a bit confusing (one "prepares" for all phases, not just the first phase; "confrontation" has aggressive interpersonal connotations not appropriate in many situations; "arousal" can disrupt anytime; not all disruptive feelings, for example "helplessness," are always associated with arousal). I prefer neutral, and parallel descriptors: pre-stress, onset-stress, mid-stress, and post-stress. Taking such a detailed examination can help people identify difficult moments when relapse is possible. For example, one person might describe the following stress situation:

> Tomorrow I'm going on a big job interview. I think about it all day and can't get it out of my mind. It keeps me up all night and I'm afraid I'll wake up tired and weary-looking. (Pre-stress) On the day of my big interview I walk up to my possible employer. I knock on the door of her office, introduce myself, and begin the interview. I start getting jittery and wonder if I will freeze up. (Onset-stress) The interview is now taking place. My interviewer asks me about my past employment as well as future goals. He asks if I have the stamina to work at this job. This last question confuses me. (Mid-stress) When the interview is over, I'm exhausted and rush home. I feel terrible and start putting myself down. I fear I've done a very bad job. (Post-stress)

The pre-stress phase refers to any period of time before the onset of the main event. Here a client is likely to be preoccupied with feelings of anticipation. In our interview example, the pre-stress phase was the day before the interview. At the onset-stress phase a client faces the beginning of a stress situation, the interview starts. In mid-stress, the stress event, the interview for example, is actually taking place. Finally, in the post-stress phase, the stress situation is over. However, some important things can still happen. Clients can, as happened in our example, needlessly worry about their performance, put themselves down, or fail to learn from mistakes. See Table 7.1 for more examples.

Develop and Deploy a SIT Rehearsal Script

Once one has a hierarchy (complete with relapse situations), the next step is to select a relaxation exercise and a good collection of reality-checking, coping, fallback, and comeback statements. See Table 7.1 for examples patterned after Meichenbaum (1985) and others.

When relaxation is used to evoke R-States targeted to helping one withdraw from stress, and defuse and desensitize anxiety, techniques such as progressive muscle relaxation and autogenic training might be appropriate. In contrast, when one desires R-States (such as Aware or Energized) to help one effectively approach and engage a potentially

TABLE 7.1   Examples of Relaxation, Reality-Checking, and Coping
Statements for Phases of a Stress Encounter

Prestress coping and relapse
"Relax!"
"Even if I can't anticipate what might happen, practicing getting into a
   problem-solving frame of mind is a good idea."
"It's normal to get tense before a stress situation."
"Let's see if I can use this stress energy productively."
"I'll set aside just 30 minutes for worrying and planning ahead."
"All I can do is change that which can be changed, and forget about the rest."
"Just keep busy, it's better than wasting time getting upset."

Onset-stress coping and relapse
"Relax!"
"It's normal to get tense just before a stress situation."
"Now's the time to do my relaxation exercise. Now take a deep breath, and relax."
"Some of this stress energy will actually help me do my best."
"I'm well-prepared, with my coping and relapse plans."
"It will be over very soon."
"Even if I get cold hands, that won't be particularly noticeable."
"What if I forget what to say! STOP! One step at a time."

Mid-stress coping and relapse
"Relax!"
"OK, it isn't the end of the world if I make a mistake."
"I can use this as an opportunity to practice dealing with stress."
"Just remember to use reason to deal with my fear."
"One step at a time—I can deal with this."
"Let's not get too personally involved."
"Let's again take a constructive, problem-solving attitude."
"Just sit back and think of all alternative courses of action, then make a choice."
"There's no need to make more out of this than is necessary."
"Don't focus on fear or anxiety, just what I have to do."
"This anxiety (or anger) is normal."
"Take care not to leap to conclusions."
"Look for the positive; don't think negative."
"Relax. Use my relaxation mini-relaxation."

Post-stress coping and relapse
"Relax!"
"Even small successes are important."
"It doesn't make sense to put myself down for gradual progress."
"In learning new skills, it's normal to have ups and downs."
"I may be upset, but I deserve a pat on the back for making an attempt to cope."
"Sure, it felt bad. But it wasn't as bad as it could be."
"This is not an absolute disaster; I'm making more out of the situation than it's
   worth."
"So, it didn't work perfectly. I can accept that."
"Next time I'll know what to expect, and can cope even better."
"It doesn't make any sense to waste time putting myself down when things
   are over."

stressful task, breathing exercises or yoga stretching might be emphasized. Mini-relaxations targeted to a particular stressor can be particularly effective.

SIT can then begin. As in simple exposure and desensitization, one
vividly images each situation, recording SUDS scores. However, attention is paid to distorted negative and coping thoughts. Specifically, for
each situation I recommend covering the following six steps (use form on
Figure 7.1) for each item on a hierarchy: As in exposure or desensitization, the client vividly imagines the details of a stress situation, including
who, what, where, and when. First describe the situation. Then:

1. *Note cues.* Think or suggest the cues that indicate that stress is beginning to build. These are cues one has determined beforehand when considering stress situation hierarchy details. Record SUDS score.

2. *Note distorted thoughts.* Think or suggest the negative distorted
thoughts one might begin to have in the stress situation. Record SUDS
score.

3. *Note maladaptive behaviors (if any).* Note any urge to avoid or escape
the stressful situation, or any behaviors that actually make the situation
worse. Record SUDS score.

4. *Stop. Relax.* Stop thinking negative thoughts (perhaps through
thought stopping) and relax using a mini-relaxation. When taught by a
counselor, the practitioner nods their head "yes" when relaxed. Record
SUDS score.

5. *Think appropriate realistic, coping thoughts, and behaviors.* Now, imagine thinking replacement thoughts that are useful and rational as well as
appropriate coping behavior. Record SUDS score.

6. *Evaluate and reward.* One thinks back over the stressful encounter
and rewards him or herself for skills that have been applied, and identifies what specific skills might be applied better. Rewards should be
immediate and relevant ("Good job! I practiced my coping strategy! I
deserve an ice cream bar"), not distant and remote ("Eventually I'll get
the job, find the right spouse, pay off my bills, etc."). Record SUDS score.

A client may choose to precede this sequence with relaxation, although
this step is optional.

A client repeats each situation (see Exposure discussion) until he or
she can rehearse it with a SUDS score no higher than 4 or 5. When this is
achieved, the sequence is repeated without initially noting distorted
thoughts and maladaptive behaviors. If appropriate, step 4 (relaxation)
may also be omitted, except in situations when relaxation is designed to
evoke R-States to prepare for encounter with a stressor (R-States Aware,
Energized) rather than withdrawal from a stressor (R-State Disengagement). If SUDS scores increase, one resumes with the entire sequence.

SITUATION Hierarchy Rank ___ Who, What, When, Where	CUE	DISTORTED THOUGHTS Omit when SUDS is less than 4 or 5 for all steps	MALADAPTIVE BEHAVIORS Omit when SUDS is less than 4 or 5 for all steps	RELAXATION Omit when SUDS is less than 4 or 5 for all steps	REALISTIC COPING THOUGHTS/ BEHAVIORS	EVALUATION AND REWARD
SUDS		SUDS	SUDS	SUDS	SUDS	SUDS

SUDS: 10 = MAXIMUM DISCOMFORT, 5 = MODERATE DISCOMFORT, 0 = NO DISCOMFORT.

FIGURE 7.1 Form for stress inoculation training (create one sheet for each of 10 situations).

The following example illustrates the six steps we have considered. A trained counselor actually describes the details to the client (details have been worked out ahead with the client).

[PRECEDE BY DESCRIBING SITUATION IN DETAIL] CUE	You can see your instructor passing out the exams. He slowly walks up and down the aisles. The clock is slowly ticking. He approaches you and hands you your exam and your heart starts to beat wildly. What is your SUDS score? [SUDS SCORE: 9]
DISTORTED THOUGHTS	You start thinking, "This is it! I'm going to fail. This exam is going to be so difficult I won't be able to finish it."
MALADAPTIVE BEHAVIOR	SUDS score? [SUDS SCORE: 9] I want to give up, turn my exam in, and leave. SUDS Score? [SUDS SCORE: 7]
STOP. RELAX	Now, think "STOP!". Imagine yourself closing your eyes. Scrunch up your shoulders real tight while taking a deep breath, and let go. Let the tension flow out. Let yourself become more and more relaxed. When you are
REALISTIC COPING THOUGHTS AND BEHAVIORS	relaxed, shake your head "yes." SUDS? [SUDS SCORE: 3] Your exam is now in front of you. You think, "This won't be so bad. I'll go through one time and just answer the easiest questions and put a little mark beside the questions that look really tough. I'll answer these last." Start answering each question that is easy. SUDS? [SUDS SCORE: 4]
REWARD & EVALUATION	When you finish the exam, you say to yourself, "Good, I got through without panicking. I remembered to just answer the easy questions first. I'm learning my coping skills." SUDS? [SUDS SCORE: 3]

These steps may initially seem a bit complex. However, they are little more than a refinement of our Cue–Response–Consequence model. However, note that the "Response" has been expanded into three parts:

Negative Response - Relaxation - Positive Response

The "negative response" includes distorted thinking and maladaptive behavior, whereas the "positive response" includes realistic coping thoughts and behavior.

SECTION 4: PROCESSES UNDERLYING REVIEW AND REHEARSAL

It should be clear that review and rehearsal strategies work in part through the application of techniques we have already learned, that is, relaxation, problem-solving, and cognitive change. In addition, four general processes may contribute to the efficacy of these approaches. First, in a safe, empathic, and supportive environment that provides reminder cues of a stressor situation, potentially disruptive hidden feelings can be brought to the surface, experienced, processed, and released. Through such *emotional insight* one "gets it off one's chest" and releases the energy-draining burden of bottled up or confused feelings of distress. Second, through *counter conditioning*, feelings of distress are replaced by feelings of relaxation. Relaxation is consistently paired with distress; eventually, stimuli that evoke distress evoke its opposite, relaxation. Third, by gently confronting a fearful stimulus, one learns that it is not as dangerous as it originally seemed. One "gets used to it," as one might get used to the constant background drone of an air conditioner. Distress weakens our *habituation*. Fourth, distress can *extinguish*. To explain, at times distress is rewarded and maintained through avoidance. For example, one might cancel a difficult confrontation with the boss, and as a result feel great relief. Avoiding the boss has been rewarded (through the good feelings of relief), and is likely to persist. Deliberately rehearsing confronting the boss deprives one of this reward, increasing the likelihood of productive (and possibly rewarding) direct encounter.

SECTION 5: WHEN TO CHOOSE EXPOSURE, DESENSITIZATION, OR STRESS INOCULATION TRAINING

The decision to choose among desensitization, exposure, or stress inoculation training depends on a variety of factors. Generally, the clinician might start with the simplest approach (exposure), and then consider approaches that are increasingly complex (desensitization, SIT). In addition, I find it useful to consider the following (See Figure 7.2):

• *Past trauma vs. future stressor.* All techniques can be applied for review or rehearsal.

	Exposure	Desensitization	SIT
Past trauma	Yes	Yes	Yes
Future stressor	Yes	Yes	Yes
Presence of initial debilitating anxiety	?	Yes	?
Chronic stressors unlikely to change	No	Yes	?/Yes
Complex problem	?	?	Yes
Deficiencies in active coping	?	?	Yes
Low initial motivation	No	Yes	No
High initial motivation	Possibly	?	Yes
History of failed coping techniques	No	Possibly	Yes
Need for professional instruction	Yes	?	Yes

FIGURE 7.2   Choosing exposure, desensitization, or stress inoculation training.

• *Presence of initial debilitating or overwhelming anxiety.* If high levels of initial anxiety prevent one from even approaching or thinking about a stressor, then desensitization is appropriate. This technique immediately reduces initial anxiety. Exposure techniques run the risk of overwhelming the client with anxiety. The complexity of SIT may also increase the risk of overwhelming anxiety.

• *Presence of chronic stressors unlikely to change.* Stress associated with chronic illness, the constant threat of terrorism, or an external stressor not likely to change as a result of active coping may respond best to desensitization deployed as an emotion-focused technique (chapter 2). As an alternative, SIT can be applied to secondary problems triggered by the chronic stressor (a chronic illness necessitating that one visit the hospital regularly for uncomfortable tests).

• *Complexity of problem.* Simple problems often respond well to relatively simple review/rehearsal strategies (exposure/desensitization) whereas more complex problems may call for SIT.

• *Presence of deficiencies in active coping.* If a client has clear deficiencies in coping (lack of problem-solving skills, propensity to engage in distorted thinking, lack of assertiveness, problems with hostility), SIT is appropriate. This approach most readily provides a way to incorporate rehearsal of specific active coping skills.

• *Degree of motivation.* Individuals with a low level of motivation to learn stress management skills may benefit most from desensitization. This approach is very easy to learn and provides strong initial reinforcements from learning relaxation. Highly motivated and educated clients may benefit most from SIT.

• *History of failed coping attempts.* Clients who have unsuccessfully tried stress management in the past may benefit from relapse prevention incorporated in SIT. To a lesser extent, desensitization may be applied, providing it is preceded by a full program of ABC Relaxation Training (chapter 4; also Smith, 1999a, 1999b, 2001). Often stress management fails because of mechanical and simplistic one-technique application of relaxation training (for example, with everyone receiving progressive muscle relaxation). ABC relaxation is an appropriate counter to such popular training failures.

• *Technique safety and need for professional instruction.* All the techniques presented here are most effective when taught by appropriately trained health professionals. Individuals may attempt desensitization on their own for relatively minor problems. A highly motivated person may try SIT. Under no conditions should a client try exposure techniques without professional guidance. This approach is often very uncomfortable to practice. Clients are tempted to terminate prematurely, minimizing effectiveness. Continued exposure to a stressor can evoke strong symptoms and negative affect, requiring professional guidance.

EXERCISES

1. Construct two simple exposure/desensitization hierarchies, one using temporal proximity and the other logical similarity as a criterion for selecting items.
2. Construct a stress inoculation hierarchy. For each step, outline what might be included. Use Figure 7.1 (make 10 copies, one for each step in the hierarchy).
3. Identify a personal stress situation in which you experienced relapse. What comeback and fallback strategies might you use?
4. Identify some distorted thoughts that can interfere with completing stress inoculation training.
5. Create a relapse situation. Generate a script.
6. In what ways can exposure techniques be centered activities involving letting go and simple, sustained focus? Include the role of R-States.
7. (FOR CLINICIANS) Construct a stress inoculation hierarchy (a full 10 pages, one for each situation) for someone else. Explain to the person that you are completing an exercise and need to obtain a complete portrait of how someone experiences stress.

Part III

Interpersonal Skills: Relationships and Stress Management

8

Assertiveness

I would like to begin with an observation: perhaps 95% of stress is inter-personal. The vast majority of problems we encounter involve, either directly or indirectly, interactions with other people. It is easy to miss this if we consider the vast popular literature of stress management texts. Major texts devote chapters to such topics as

Occupational stress
The stress of being a woman
The stress of being a college student
The stress of being in a family
The stress of growing old
The stress of being a racial/ethnic/religious/sexual orientation minority

Interpersonal stress might be slipped in, one chapter among many. I think this is a mistake. Careful consideration of each of these and other topics reveals their interpersonal core. For example, job stress is an amal-gam of many factors, including poor work conditions not effectively addressed by others in charge, conflict with coworkers and superiors, excessive or vague job responsibilities expected by others, and so on. In other words, most job stress involves our relationships with people. Take another example, the stress of being a college student. Here again we find interpersonal problems: dating, dealing with unfair professors, finding and coping with roommates, getting help from others, and so on. Most stress is interpersonal.

What about some apparently impersonal stressors, such as recovering from cancer, dealing with a home-destroying fire, or managing chronic back pain? If we look, again we find a major interpersonal component. Obviously each has an impersonal element, such as diet, medication, and surgery (cancer), recovering damaged property, finding a place to live (fire), and possible painkillers (back pain). But just as important is the role of people. The cancer survivor may have to learn to relate to others in a way that is conducive to generating positive, healing states of mind, R-States (chapter 4). He or she may need to negotiate changes in work responsibilities. Help from others may be solicited. Similarly, the fire victim may need to deal with bank loan officers for financing, deal with upset family members, and find social support in friends and relatives. The pain patient may well take painkillers, but often they are not completely effective. She may have to address interpersonal stress that aggravates pain.

If stress usually involves people, then it follows that most specific applications of stress management are also interpersonal. In terms of our four pillars of stress management, one learns to relate to others in a way conducive to: experiencing a full range of R-States (with relationships that are "happy," "peaceful," "thankful and loving," etc.), solving interpersonal problems, productively checking the reality of distorted cognitions about others, and systematically reviewing past interpersonal traumas and rehearsing for future encounters. There is a term that encompasses most interpersonal applications: "assertiveness."

Assertiveness is a popular topic in stress management. This chapter provides an overview that summarizes and integrates points frequently made and repeated by others (Alberti, 1977; Alberti & Emmons, 1982; Bedell & Lennox, 1997; Bower & Bower, 1991; Jakubowski & Lange, 1978).

ASSERTIVENESS (vs. PASSIVITY, AGGRESSIVENESS, AND PASSIVE-AGGRESSIVENESS)

To be assertive is to honestly and effectively express one's wants, thoughts, and feelings while empathically recognizing and respecting the wants, thoughts, and feelings of others. Assertive skills are often seen as most likely to prevent and reduce stress. The assertive person is more likely to directly solve a problem, achieve a satisfying compromise, and not be distracted by maladaptive and distorted thinking. An assertive person is also more likely to experience deep relaxation, undistracted by unresolved conflict and desire.

Traditionally, assertiveness is contrasted with passivity and aggressiveness. To this I add passive-aggressiveness. The passive person fails to express his or her wants, thoughts, and feelings. One keeps to oneself, unheard and unrecognized. Problems are left unresolved, and wants unfulfilled. The aggressive person expresses wants, thoughts, and feelings, but without empathically respecting the wants, thoughts, and feelings of others. The short-term result of aggression may well be fulfillment of a want or reduction of certain types of stress; however, there is often a short-term and long-term cost. Finally, a special type of nonassertive behavior should be noted. The passive-aggressive individual does not express his or her wants, thoughts, and feelings. However, they do express aggression indirectly (so they don't have to assertively assume responsibility).

EXAMPLES OF ASSERTIVE, PASSIVE, AGGRESSIVE, AND PASSIVE-AGGRESSIVE BEHAVIOR

People often think they are assertive, when in fact they're not. It can be helpful to consider some examples to refine one's ability to differentiate assertive and nonassertive behavior. Consider the following.

The Dishes

James and Dale have been roommates for over a year. They have arranged to divide living chores, with James doing the dishes every other day. It has been over a week and James has not done his work. With dishes piling up, Dale finally decides to have a few words.

ASSERTIVE DALE:	"James, I thought you agreed we would share the chores, with you doing dishes every other day. I understand this is not a pleasant job for you, and I don't like it either. But let's talk about our chores. For the last week the dishes haven't been done. I'm feeling frustrated, like you aren't carrying your weight. I would feel a lot better about our arrangement if we could come to an understanding we both like."
AGGRESSIVE DALE:	"James, do the dishes. You're just lazy and irresponsible."
PASSIVE DALE:	"James, I wonder if we could, you know, be a little more cooperative here. I know you're busy, and that's fine."
PASSIVE-AGGRESSIVE DALE:	"OK, don't do the dishes. Well, I just can't seem to find a place to store all my extra junk. Your bedroom will do nicely."

Asking for a Raise

Susan has been working as an accountant at a real-estate firm for nearly 2 years. Although she signed on with the unwritten understanding that there would be a yearly raise, and a bonus when business is good, she has received no raise. Business has indeed been very good, Susan's work evaluations have been excellent, and others have received raises. She decides to have a meeting with her supervisor.

ASSERTIVE SUSAN:	"I would like to talk about my raise this year. I believe my performance has been fine and the corporation has been making money. I think under those conditions a raise would be appropriate. And I was very confused when I received no raise."
AGGRESSIVE SUSAN:	"This is unacceptable. I get no raise; clearly you selfish pigs do not appreciate all the work I have been doing. I just can't take the abuse here."
PASSIVE SUSAN:	"I wonder if we could talk about my work here, if you don't mind. I hope I've been doing okay. I really like working here with you. This is really such a wonderful place."
PASSIVE-AGGRESSIVE SUSAN:	"I really like the way you efficiently run this company. You clearly save money by not giving raises to staff you don't respect."

Feeling Left Out of a Conversation

Roberta, Georgette, and Ann have been chatting over a cup of coffee Saturday afternoon. Georgette and Ann have monopolized the conversation, talking about their mutual interests, frustrations, boyfriends, and so on. Whenever Roberta attempts to say something, her two friends say a few polite words, and then resume talking about their interests. After 20 minutes, Roberta feels left out and wants to bring the issue up.

ASSERTIVE ROBERTA:	"Hey, girlfriends, I feel a little left out here. I enjoy listening to what you've got to say, but I really would like to hear what you've got to say about my latest date. I'm getting frustrated just keeping it to myself and not telling anyone. My turn."
AGGRESSIVE ROBERTA:	"You ladies are always talking about yourselves. Don't you care about anyone else? I feel like a worthless thing."
PASSIVE ROBERTA:	"Excuse me . . . Excuse me . . . That was real interesting . . . ah . . . uh."

PASSIVE-AGGRESSIVE ROBERTA: "Oh, don't mind me. Just keep on talking to each other. It doesn't bother me, really. You clearly have something more important to talk about. I don't matter, really."

COSTS AND BENEFITS

To learn assertive skills increases one's choices. Using problem-solving strategies (chapter 5), one can weigh the costs and benefits of assertiveness, passivity, aggressiveness, and passive-aggressiveness, and then decide what to do. However, all texts on assertiveness claim that the costs of nonassertiveness typically outweigh the benefits. Assertive people are more likely to get what they want, enlist the cooperation and help of others, enjoy satisfying relationships, and have a higher opinion of themselves.

Passive (and passive-aggressive) people, because they keep their wants, thoughts, and feelings to themselves, are more likely to be frustrated and not get what they want. They are more likely to be manipulated and injured by others. The passive person is more likely to experience stress and distorted thinking, and less likely to resolve stressful problems. As a result, he or she may have difficulties with deep relaxation exercises and not experience the benefits of relaxation states of mind in everyday life.

Aggressive people may temporarily get what they want and feel satisfied and powerful. Others are more likely to feel resentful and not cooperative, relationships are injured, and some wants may not be fulfilled. Long-term problem-solving is not enhanced and self-serving distorted thinking may persist. Generally, the aggressive (and passive-aggressive) person carries an additional burden of physical and psychological tension that can interfere with both practicing a relaxation exercise and enjoying relaxation throughout work and leisure. See Table 8.1 for a list of many of the costs and benefits frequently suggested (Alberti & Emmons, 1982; Bedell & Lennox, 1997; Bower & Bower, 1991; Jakubowski & Lange, 1978; Peterson, 2000).

NONVERBAL BEHAVIORS

One's wants, thoughts, and feelings can be communicated nonverbally. Developing the ability to read such subtle cues can help the nonassertive person detect when they are being passive or aggressive. There are three types of nonverbal behaviors to consider: voice; eye movements and facial expression; and body movements, gestures, and postures. See Table 8.2 for a sample of some nonverbal behaviors many others (Alberti &

TABLE 8.1   Costs and Benefits of Assertive and Nonassertive Behavior

Assertive	
Possible costs	Possible benefits
Requires honest effort to consider one's actual wants, thoughts, and feelings	Perhaps more likely to achieve one's wants and resolve issues
One must forgo the short-term satisfaction of "getting even"	Less likely to offend others and provoke needless hostility
One must forgo the short-term satisfaction of avoiding an issue	More likely to maintain friendships and working, adult relationships
Requires effort to attend to and respect empathically the wants, thoughts, and feelings of others	Enhanced feeling of self-esteem and personal effectiveness
One may have to deal with the assertive response of the other person	
One may have to consider compromise of what one wants	

Passive/Passive-aggressive	
Possible costs	Possible benefits
Failure to get what one wants	Avoid temporary discomfort of honestly stating what one wants, thinks, feels
Failure to express one's wants, thoughts, and feelings	Not having to exert the effort to articulate wants, thoughts, feelings
Misunderstanding from other people	Perhaps can get others to take care of one
Relationships suffer	
Open to manipulation by others	
Others see one as whining	
Lowered self-esteem	

Aggressive/Passive-aggressive	
Possible costs	Possible benefits
Invites hostility from others	Temporarily get what one wants
Relationships suffer	Temporary feeling of power and control
Others see one as selfish, manipulative	Temporary confirmation of personal distortion
May "burn bridges" and reduce possibility of getting what one wants in the future	
Reduces likelihood of cooperation from others	

TABLE 8.2 Assertive, Passive/Passive-Aggressive, and Aggressive Nonverbal Behavior

Eye contact and facial expression		
Assertive	Passive/Passive/Aggressive	Aggressive

Eye-to-eye contact direct
Expressive
Shows appropriate
  emotion
	Avoiding looking at other
	Nervous blinking, looking
	  at watch
	Inappropriate and defensive
	  smiling, laughing, giggling
	Tension signs of feelings
	  "bottled up" (biting lips,
	  clenching jaws, chewing,
	  clearing throat, wrinkling
	  forehead)
		Staring down
		Looking into distance
		  (bored, irritated)
		Squinting
		Clenching jaws
		Shaking head
		Furrowing brow
		Frowning, showing
		  teeth

Voice		
Assertive	Passive/Passive/Aggressive	Aggressive

Normal and appropriate
  volume, inflection,
  and speed
Sound of voice
  consistent with
  what is being said
	Speaking too quietly,
	  whispering, mumbling
	Too slow or fast
	"Whining," "hinting," tone
	  suggesting of themes not
	  discussed
	Pauses
		Too fast or loud
		Pauses or abrupt
		  interruption of
		  other person

Posture, gestures, and movements		
Assertive	Passive/Passive/Aggressive	Aggressive

Relaxed, natural looking,
  matches and
  appropriately
  accentuates content
  of what is being said.
Sits or stand upright,
  attentive to other
  person
Appropriate distance
  from other person
	Unnecessary "nervous"
	  movements such as
	  fidgeting
	Complete lack of movement;
	  frozen
	Faces away from other person
	Stands too far away
	Slumps, bowed, sloped
	  shoulders, hand behind
	  back
	Wringing or holding hands
	Shaking head (in agreement)
		Unnecessary
		  distracting
		Movements such as
		  fidgeting, looking at
		  clock, adjusting tie
		Shaking head (in
		  disagreement)
		Pointing, making fist
		Hands on hips
		Stands too close

Emmons, 1982; Bedell & Lennox, 1997; Bower & Bower, 1991; Jakubowski & Lange, 1978) have noted. Many experts, including Alberti and Emmons (1982) and Jakubowski and Lange (1978) have a useful way of describing realistic beliefs supportive of assertiveness: *assertive rights*. Some of their rights include (supplemented with a few of my own):

Assertive Rights (Beliefs)

You have the right to dignity and self-respect.
You have the right not to feel guilty.
You have the right to say no.
You have the right to have and express feelings, even those that others might not approve of.
You have the right to change your mind.
You have the right to ask for help and for what you want.
You have the right to be less than what others expect of you.

In addition, various distorted beliefs may contribute to passive, aggressive, and passive/aggressive behavior. Some noted by various writers of assertiveness (Alberti & Emmons, 1982; Bedell & Lennox, 1997; Bower & Bower, 1991; Jakubowski & Lange, 1978) include:

Distorted Passive Beliefs

You must have the approval of others.
If you are honest with others, they will retaliate.
Things will get better on their own.
It's really not that important.
Asking for something is selfish and needlessly inconveniences others. It is better just to keep your wants to yourself.
You are always responsible for the hurt feelings of others.
People who hold in their own wants, thoughts, and feelings are more likable.
You should feel terribly guilty if something you say happens to bother other people.
Others can usually figure out what you want, think, or feel.
The best way to respect others is not to make waves and express yourself.
The world is a dangerous place, it is best to keep quiet.
If you express your feelings, others will think you are too aggressive or misunderstand your intentions.

Distorted Aggressive Beliefs

People who do or say things that end up hurting you do so deliberately, or are evil.

You must win in order for others to accept you.

The world is a dangerous, hostile place where one always has to be on guard.

People who don't come on strong aren't listened to.

If you compromise, you won't get what you want.

People won't take you seriously, or think you are a real man (or woman) unless you are tough.

Distorted Passive-Aggressive Beliefs

If you express your anger indirectly, others will get your point.

If you can't get what you want, get even.

It is dangerous to express anger in such a way that you can be identified.

It is better to pretend that things are OK, and hurt the other person indirectly.

If people are punished, they will figure out on their own what they did wrong.

It is cool not to say what you want, but cause trouble for others who cause problems.

Just in case your anger and frustration is not justified, it is better to express it in such a way that others won't know who is responsible.

In chapter 6 we considered three categories of distorted thinking: unrealistic desires or expectations, exaggerated negative reaction, and fatalism and helplessness. Each can contribute to nonassertive behavior. A passive person might have the unrealistic expectation that he or she should be perfect in order to make friends. An aggressive person might respond to a perceived insult with an exaggerated negative reaction and catastrophize. A passive-aggressive person who wants to ask someone else to change an offensive behavior may feel helpless, and act out with an indirect and hostile hint. Any of the distorted beliefs in the Smith Irrational Beliefs Inventory (Table 6.1) can contribute to a lack of assertiveness.

EMPATHY, SHYNESS AND SOCIAL
ANXIETY, CONFLICT

We can now take a deeper look at assertiveness and stress. In chapters to come we will consider three types of assertive skills. When the focus is primarily on the other person, and understanding what he or she wants, thinks, or feels, the assertive task is *empathic listening and responding*. When the focus is primarily on oneself, and one's anxieties over interacting with others or doing things in public, we consider *shyness and social anxiety*. Finally, in *conflict* situations, the focus is on differences between the wants, thoughts, and feelings of oneself and another.

EXERCISES

1. Think of examples in your own life, or examples you have observed, that illustrate assertiveness, passivity, aggressiveness, and passive-aggressiveness. In a group, consider if these categorizations are correct. Often assertive and aggressive replies are confused.
2. Select five examples of assertive behavior, five passive, five aggressive, and five passive-aggressive. What nonverbal behavior did you observe for each?
3. For each of the above examples, list the costs and benefits of the behavior.
4. In your experience, what distorted thoughts contributed to nonassertive behavior? Passive behavior? Aggressive behavior? Passive-aggressive behavior?
5. Generate a realistic response to each distorted thought the book, or you, have associated with assertive, passive, aggressive, and passive/aggressive behavior.
6. In a group, members select an interpersonal situation to act out. Other group members identify if it is assertive, passive, aggressive, or passive-aggressive. Other group members discuss their reasons, including what nonverbal behaviors were observed. Discuss the costs and benefits of each behavior. Also discuss how nonassertive behavior might be more assertive.
7. In a group, select a nonassertive situation role-played in Question 6. Discuss how it might be acted out more assertively. Then act it out and review.

9

Empathic Listening

Empathic listening is perhaps the forgotten stress management skill. However, much interpersonal stress can be minimized and reduced if one clearly understands the other person's experienced feelings, as well as their wants, thoughts, and behaviors. We have already considered clarification of one's own needs and priorities in previous chapters, specifically in the context of unfulfilled wants (chapter 5) and distorted and unrealistic thinking (chapter 6). In future chapters we will consider the process of articulating one's wants in terms of shyness, social anxiety, and conflict. In this chapter we change our focus from oneself to other participants in a stress situation. What does the other person feel? What do they want and think? In addition, what is their perception of their own behavior (what do they think they're doing)?

SECTION 1: EMPATHY AND ASSERTIVE COPING

Assertiveness without empathy is incomplete and can create problems. Consider the following exchange. Chris and Tony have been dating for a year and are engaged to be married. Recently they both went to a party together. Tony spent most of the time talking with her other friends she had not seen for a while. Chris stood alone and was upset. In this version, Chris does not recognize Tony's perspective.

> CHRIS: "At the party I felt abandoned and alone. You spent your time talking with other people. I found myself wondering if you were dumping me or trying to get back at me for something I did. Was it something I did? Is our relationship in trouble? I feel stuck and confused."

In the following version, Chris makes some attempt to understand Tony's thoughts, feelings, and wants.

CHRIS: "At the party I noticed you talking to some other
                  people. It seemed like you were enjoying old friends
                  you hadn't seen for a long time and got really
                  involved in "catching up" with each other's lives.
                  But I felt left out, abandoned, and alone. I even found
                  myself wondering if you were dumping me or trying
                  to get back at me for something I did. Let's talk."

Note how Chris's attempt at empathy enabled him to gain perspective
over his own feelings of abandonment and confusion over his friend's
motives. The first example lacks this empathic awareness. Lacking empathic information, Chris is more likely to entertain distorted and catastrophic
thinking ("Is our relationship in trouble?") and less likely to approach his
concern with productive problem-solving ("I feel stuck and confused.
Let's talk.").

Generally, the effort of trying to understand another's perspective in
a stressful encounter increases the likelihood of acquiring important
information and reduces the chances of isolated distorted thinking. It
is also much more likely to communicate to the other person a will-
ingness to resolve problems in an mature assertive manner, rather than
through aggressive attack or passive withdrawal. Indeed our own
research indicates that empathy is an important part of negotiation and
problem-solving.

SECTION 2: CUE–RESPONSE–CONSEQUENCES

Much has been written on empathy; the ideas of this chapter are modifi-
cations and integrations of suggestions presented in countless texts of
counseling and psychotherapy, most notably those of Bedell and Lennox
(1997), Bohart and Greenberg (1997), Egan (1998), Meichenbaum (1985),
and Watson (2002).

Empathy is accurately understanding a person's feelings, as well as
their wants, thoughts, and perceived behaviors, and clearly communicating this understanding. One begins by observing the responses of
another, however, a full empathic observation has three parts, recognition
of the Cue, the Response, and (when possible), the Consequence to the
other person, or C–R–C. Consider the following interaction:

OTHER PERSON: "All these new assignments at the job. When I look
               at my desk, I don't know if I can continue working at
               this pace. And I sit and do nothing and feel awful."

LISTENER: "You feel overwhelmed because of all the new work.
               You are beginning to wonder if you have it in you
               to do it, and end up sitting. Then you feel bad about
               yourself."

Here the cue is "the new work" and the noted response is "sitting and doing nothing" (and possibly the thought "I don't know if I can continue working at this place."). And the perceived consequence is "feeling bad about yourself." Note that the listener's empathic observation notes the entire C—R–C chain. In sum, a listener is most likely to give a full empathic response that notes all facets of C-R–C if he or she uses the simple formula (Egan, 1998):

"You feel and think _____ because _____."

SECTION 3: WHAT TO LOOK FOR WHEN MAKING EMPATHIC INFERENCES

Initially, empathy should stick fairly closely to the facts and what the person is stating. There are times one must make reasonable guesses concerning affect and content that may be hidden beneath the surface. There are several types of information that can be used (Bedell & Lennox, 1997; Egan, 1998).

Nonverbal Language

A skilled listener must also be a skilled observer. People present a wealth of nonverbal information through facial expressions, posture, gestures, voice quality, physiological responses (tics, sweating, breathing hard), and general appearance (grooming, dress). Sometimes such nonverbal cues reinforce what the person is talking about:

OTHER PERSON: (MAKING A FIST, LEANING FORWARD, SPEAKING LOUD AND FAST): "I'm really angry with my landlord for increasing the rent."

At other times nonverbal cues are either inconsistent with what is being said, or have a message of their own:

OTHER PERSON: (SLOUCHING, LOOKING DOWN, SPEAKING IN QUIET, MEEK VOICE): "I'm really angry with my landlord for increasing the rent."

One type of empathic inference is to simply report to the person the message you think his or her nonverbal language is conveying:

OTHER PERSON: (BITING NAILS, SPEAKING SOFTLY, LOOKING DOWN): "Maybe I should talk to my professor about taking the test over."

LISTENER: "I sense from your posture that you are a bit nervous about talking to your professor."

What One Might Experience in Similar Circumstances

When people leave certain things unsaid, it can be up to you to fill in the blanks. One way of making reasonable inferences is to think about what you might experience in similar circumstances:

OTHER PERSON: "I've been dating Jill for nearly a year. She tells me I'm the only one she's dating. I thought things were getting pretty serious. Then last week I saw her going to a movie with another woman. I had suggested that we see the movie together."

LISTENER: "I'm not sure what you're feeling, but I think I would be confused in such a situation and wonder why she's out with another person."

Drawing from the Other Person's Past

People may leave unstated important facts and feelings that become clear when seen in the context of what has happened in similar past stress situations:

OTHER PERSON: "I blew up at work again. Those people just make me so angry. I don't know what's going on. Who do they think they are?"

LISTENER: "I hear your anger, but I'm not quite sure where it's coming from. I can't help recalling the last three or four times you blew up at work you discovered someone else was doing your job for you."

Drawing from What Others Would Likely Experience in Similar Circumstances

OTHER PERSON: "I was at the doctor's office getting special tests for my chest pains. When the tests were over, I asked him if I was OK. He said he didn't know and would let me know next week if I had to take more tests. I felt really messed up."

LISTENER: "I think being left up in the air about important health questions would make most people a little anxious."

Summarizing Briefly What the Person Has Already Said

People can share a wealth of information, and then feel confused about what they're feeling. One way of helping is to pull together the most important points:

OTHER PERSON: "I'm waiting in line at the grocery store. This man pushes in front of me without apologizing. Before I could say a thing, he's out. On this road, this woman behind me keeps honking her horn. I get really peeved. She makes a fist and yells at me to speed up. My boss dumps a big report on my desk and says, "Do this." He leaves without explaining anything."

LISTENER: "I notice you've been describing a number of times when people irritate you by being rude and inconsiderate."

Considering What the Other Person Is Saying in Terms of the Basic Feelings of Fear, Happiness, Anger, and Sadness

Bedell and Lennox (1997) have a useful suggestion for those practicing empathic understanding of feelings. When another person communicates a feeling that seems confusing or unclear, one can attempt to determine which of four basic feelings—anxiety, depression, anger, or happiness—it resembles. Often this requires considering previous sources of information we have discussed. And recall (chapter 5) that anxiety often suggests withdrawal in face of threat, anger approach and confrontation of a provocation, and depression, lack of reinforcement, giving up, and inactivity. For example:

OTHER PERSON: "I feel very upset about breaking up with my boyfriend. He had no right just to walk away from me without explaining his feelings. Just wait until I run into him at school!"

LISTENER: "You seem to be quite irritated at your boyfriend (Infers irritation from the approach threat, 'Just wait until I run into him at school')."

OTHER PERSON: "I feel very out of it. My kids say they don't like me and want to run away. My wife isn't talking to me. I don't know what to do. I just feel like going into the basement den and vegetating."

LISTENER: "You seem a little blue and down and out. Almost as though important people in your life aren't with you. (Infers depression from lack of reinforcement and behaviors of withdrawal.)

OTHER PERSON: "I have my big job interview tomorrow. I feel really jittery about it. I tried to get the same job last year and was turned down. I really wonder if the interviewer is going to criticize me for being too pushy. I would rather just stay home."

LISTENER: "You seem a little fearful about this interview, given the uncertainties and possibility of threat." (Infers fear from described threat and withdrawal.)

SECTION 4: EMPATHIC AND NONEMPATHIC RESPONDING

It can be helpful to keep in mind a number of "empathic prompts," or phrases that encourage people to clarify and explore feeling and content. It is important not to mechanically present prompts as questions, but put them in your own words. Meichenbaum (1985) has suggested the following:

"Correct me if I am wrong, but what I hear you saying is . . ."

"I am not sure if I quite understood; can we go over that one more time?"

"I am wondering in what ways your becoming stressed in situation ____ is like your becoming stressed in situation ____?"

"On the one hand I hear you saying ____ and on the other hand I hear you saying ____. I wonder how these two things go together."

"You seem to be telling me ____. Am I correct in assuming that?"

"I get the feeling that ____. Is that the way you see it?"

Sometimes people think they are empathic when they are not. Empathy is often confused with sympathy. Sympathy reflects how one feels *about* another person. "I feel sad that you were hurt" is sympathetic, whereas "I sense you are hurt" is empathic. Many experts (Bohart & Greenberg, 1997; Egan, 1998; Watson, 2002) have suggested long lists of nonempathic substitutes. I find it useful to think of three types of such responses: lecturing, sincere nonempathy, and near empathy. I would like to emphasize that there may indeed be a time and place for most of these responses; however, if an empathic response is appropriate and desired, the following do not count.

Lecturing: Focusing Not on the Other Person's Feeling, But on Some Point or Explanation You Want to Make

Advising

"You should call your wife up and talk things over."

"Have you considered asking your parents for a loan?"

Interpreting

"Of course you are having difficulty solving the problem. Your depression is lowering the level of brain serotonin and interfering with your ability to think."

"I understand your problems getting a job. Today's recession in your business sector has reduced demand for workers with your skill background, often requiring lateral or downward mobility."

Psychoanalyzing

"Your anxiety about dating men suggests to me that you are confused about certain sexual issues."

"That fact that you are angry that your mother asked you to visit could mean that you have deep attachments to your mother and are unwilling to let go."

Judging

"It was not right to steal from your younger brother."

"I think that getting into an argument created more problems than it solved."

Preaching

"It is because of your past sins (or bad karma) that you are having these problems."

"If you only had enough faith, this would not be a problem for you."

Mechanically Stating Cliches

"Remember, Rome was not built in a day."

"Love conquers all."

Philosophizing and Mystifying

"You are an Aquarius. That means you can expect to get depressed from time to time. You are very sensitive."

"I have psychic powers and can see that you are struggling with the Dark Forces. But your inner light will emerge when you accept them."

Sincere Nonempathy: Saying Something That May Be Caring, Supportive, or Well-Meaning, But Isn't Really Empathy

Giving Sympathy

"I know how bad it is to be depressed. I get depressed myself."

"I really feel sorry about your loss. It really upsets me."

Pitying, Humoring

"That must hurt so bad. I feel sorry for you."

"You poor thing."

Interrogating/Interviewing

"You couldn't sleep last night because of the test? How often do you lose sleep? Do you lose sleep the entire night? Are you sure you don't drink a lot of coffee before bed? I know that will keep me up every time!"

"The cop asked you for your driver's license? Was he a state trooper? Is this the first time you've been stopped for speeding? How many traffic tickets do you have?"

Inappropriate Sharing of Personal Affection or Positive Feeling Towards the Other Person (While Ignoring Their Feelings)

OTHER PERSON: "I was working on this project at work and my coworker just came in and took over. Without any explanation, she said, 'I can do this,' and started doing my work."

LISTENER: "I want you to know that I still care for you very much."

OTHER PERSON: "It's nearly midnight and my teen daughter is already a half hour late. She is supposed to be home now. I really hope she is OK. A lot of very bad things can happen to teens out in the big city."

LISTENER: "Jesus is with you."

Denying Feeling

"Don't worry. It will go away."

"Your problem isn't so bad. Look at all the troubles other people have."

Near-Empathy: Coming Close to an Underlying Feeling, But Still Missing It

Missing the Point While Saying Something That Is Generally True

OTHER PERSON: "I am getting out of this relationship. He's hurt me enough. I don't need the pain. I wonder if I should just throw in the towel and quit."

LISTENER: "I sense your frustration. Frustration can sometimes lead to aggression and irritation."

OTHER PERSON: "I thought I would get that promotion. I really planned for it. Now it seems like my life is on hold. I'm like a little puppy lost in the woods."

LISTENER: "Boy, you're angry. It's not unusual for someone who is so unfairly rejected at work to feel angry."

Narrowly Focusing on a Minor or Irrelevant Point

"You say you're upset over the bad job review you received. Well, was it right at the beginning of the day?"

"Okay, so she doesn't want to go out with you after all. Were you so preoccupied that you missed the attractive number at the end of the hall?"

Repeating the Obvious (Parroting)

OTHER PERSON: "I feel nervous and upset."

LISTENER: "You feel nervous and upset."

OTHER PERSON: "My mother doesn't know I'm married. She just called and announced she was coming to visit me, and my wife lives with me. She will find out!"

LISTENER: "You are concerned that your mother might discover you're married."

Getting the Wrong Hidden Feeling

OTHER PERSON: "I'm all tied up inside. She called me a 'fool' in front of my friends and all I could do was clench my jaws."

LISTENER: "I sense how sad and depressed you must feel over this rejection."

OTHER PERSON: "No one seems to like me. Every day I go home alone with no one to talk to. I just sit down and sulk."

LISTENER: "The world is treating you very bad. You just want to get even."

Being Vague and Imprecise

"You were describing how you were so angry you felt like punching your roommate out. You really felt messed up."

"Your diagnosis of cancer is a real concern and I understand why you would say that life seems hopeless and bleak. I sense you feel very down."

Professing Understanding When One Doesn't Understand

"Yes, yes, I know what you're talking about."

"I understand perfectly."

There is clearly a place for some of the responses that do not fit our definition of empathy. However, when nonempathic attempts at helping are inappropriate, they can have their costs. Inappropriate nonempathy leads to confusion and feelings of misunderstanding. One might think they should understand what the listener is saying, even if it doesn't make sense. Nonempathy can distract from productive problem-solving or reality-checking efforts. One might feel pushed or overwhelmed, making a problem worse. Nonempathy can contribute to interpersonal distance, mistrust, and anger, increasing the possibility of future misunderstanding.

Empathy can be communicated by speech characteristics and nonverbal behavior (Watson, 2002). Empathic speech is not hurried or rapid. One does not interrupt or immediately jump in during moments of silence, but gives the other person time to reflect and consider what to say. Voice tone communicates interest and at times emotional involvement, rather than boredome, lack of interest, or analytic detachment. The empathic individual is more likely to look directly at the other person and maintain eye contact. He or she may lean forward in a chair, rather than sit back in a relaxed position. Legs and arms are open, rather than crossed.

People are often good observers of empathic and nonempathic behavior. When listened to with empathy, the other person is likely to say such things as "I feel understood," "you are with him," "I can trust that even if you miss a point, you'll try hard to get it right," "I sense you know what it's like to be me," and "you understand." When people have helpers who are not particularly empathic, they are more likely to complain: "I don't feel you are with me or know how I feel," "you aren't hearing me out," "I wonder if you really care," "you seem not to be paying attention to what I say." The best judge of empathy is the person to whom it is directed.

SECTION 5: EMPATHY AND GENDLIN'S FOCUSING

One way of understanding empathy, and to clarify the costs of well-meant nonempathic responses, is to consider Gendlin's notion of "focusing" (chapter 5). Focusing begins when a person shares a vague statement of a feeling or problem, for example:

"I feel messed up."

"I feel upset."

One attends to this feeling without trying to analyze, figure out, or eliminate it. Instead, one simply attends, and waits for the "gist" or "felt meaning." Someone focusing on "feeling upset" may, after a few minutes, discover a hidden feeling, "I feel alone, without friends."

Empathy is a way of helping another person focus. One nonanalytically focuses on the other person's problem, and suggests what feeling, or felt meaning, might be *just beneath the surface*. Often this "gist" may be clear to you, but not to the other person. For example, a person may make a fist, clench his teeth, and loudly state "I feel totally confused and crazy about my husband abandoning me that way." A listener, noting the body language and tone of voice, as well as the logic of the situation (abandonment), suspects anger is the felt meaning just below the stated feelings of confusion and craziness. So an empathic response might be: "I sense your frustration and anger."

SECTION 6: OPEN-ENDED, PROBLEM-SOLVING, AND REALITY-CHECKING EMPATHY

Open-ended empathy involves hearing the person out, that is, trying to accurately understand and reflect the gist of whatever they have to say. Such listening enables the person to articulate hidden feelings and begin to develop a good working relationship with another person. It provides an opportunity to gain an objective impression of the other person's side of the problem.

Often when one shares one's experiences, they provide an abundance of information. Indeed, the skilled listener directs focus, attends selectively, and does not get diverted with irrelevant detail (Ivey, Ivey, & Simek-Morgan, 1977). In addition, several different empathic understandings may apply to the same utterance; here, the listener has a choice of what to reflect. I suggest two options in addition to open-ended empathy: problem-solving empathy, and reality-checking empathy.

Problem-Solving Empathy

Often, an empathic discussion shifts focus to two types of questions:

- How does the person *define* his or her problem? What does he or she want? What are their feelings about this problem and the process of defining it?
- How is the person trying to *solve* their problem? What are their feelings about the solutions considered and the process of developing them?

These questions illustrate *problem-solving empathy*. At one level, one listens to affect and content (what they are feeling and why). At another level one listens to the person attempting to define, figure out, and solve his or her problem. In terms of our framework presented earlier, one listens for: cues (early warning signs, critical moments), the problematic response (goals, missing behaviors, negative behaviors), and consequences (costs, benefits). One reflects back observed problem-defining and solution-defining efforts.

It is important to recognize the distinction between open-ended and problem-solving empathy. We can see the differences in the following examples of an unemployed man who is having considerable difficulty finding work:

UNEMPLOYED MAN:	"I keep looking through the want ads, day after day. Each day I apply for at least five or six jobs. I usually get one interview a week. But I never get the job. The jobs just aren't there. I feel terrible: I've been stuck in this rut for nearly a year and am going nowhere."
LISTENER (open-ended empathy):	"I can understand how frustrating it must be to find no jobs out there."
LISTENER (problem-solving empathy):	"You've been trying the want-ad strategy for nearly a year and are finding it just isn't panning out. This is really frustrating."

UNEMPLOYED MAN:	"What should I do? I feel so up in the air. I could call up my relatives for some leads. Or maybe talk to my old employer. Or maybe use some of my savings to go to college to learn some new job skills. I just don't know what's the best for me, and what's a dead-end street."
LISTENER (open-ended empathy):	"You feel a bit helpless, not knowing what will and will not work."
LISTENER (problem-solving empathy):	"You're starting to sort out what you could do, the pluses and minuses. You feel a bit helpless not knowing the right answer at this time."

Note that in these examples, open-ended and problem solving empathy identify feeling and content. However, the problem-solving listener wants to know how the person is trying to define and solve the problem.

Open-ended empathy tends to treat all content equally, attempting to reflect the primary content and feeling. Problem-solving empathy listens for what is specific, concrete, and realistic. Irrelevant detail, conjecture, and venting of feeling is either ignored or put in its appropriate context. The goal once again is to listen to people as they attempt to effectively figure out and solve problems. We can see this difference in emphasis in our continuing example of the unemployed man:

UNEMPLOYED MAN:	"I had a job interview last week. I had hoped it would help me solve my employment problem, but I was turned down. Damn it! I think everyone is out to get me. I just don't have what it takes to be successful at anything. I buy the wrong newspaper. I'm late for my appointment with you. I'm a loser. It gets so I feel like banging the table."

LISTENER (open-ended empathy):   "You feel really angry and frustrated when things seem to be going against you."

LISTENER (problem-solving empathy):   "That job interview seemed like a good bet. When you were turned down, you got really angry and frustrated that this idea didn't work."

Problem-solving empathy continues the process of enabling the person to express feelings and develop rapport. In addition, it subtly directs the person towards defining problems in a useful way and searching out solutions. More generally, it begins the process of helping a person discover sources of hope and optimism that are the foundation of the problem-solving frame of mind.

Reality-Checking Empathy

Empathy can also focus on reality-testing as discussed in our chapter on cognitive techniques (chapter 6). Here, in addition to listening to underlying content and feelings, one also attempts to highlight realistic fact and evaluation, and differentiate them from possible distortion.

UNEMPLOYED MAN: "Maybe I should approach my job interviews differently. I've been waiting for employers to call. You know, I could get a list of job openings, and then make an appointment to see the supervisor in person before sending in my application. That would really take guts! I can't do that, I would feel like a fool. What if they simply refuse to see me, after I get all dressed up and go all out? I couldn't take it, I would feel down and out and withdraw for a month. Too much could go wrong. I don't want to take the chance."

LISTENER (open-ended empathy):

"You are concerned that even after being careful and cautious you might feel like a fool and get depressed."

LISTENER (empathic reality-checking):

"You've identified something you could do, make an appointment, that is one option of many (realistic fact). Since you've never done this before, you're not sure how it would go. You start catastrophizing (observation of cognitive distortion)."

EXERCISES

1. Over the week observe others interacting. Note which encounters are empathic and which are not. Explain.
2. In a role-play situation, one person describes a problem, while another responds with empathy. Others in the group evaluate how the response was empathic, and how it might be improved.
3. One of the first steps in learning empathy is differentiating empathic from nonempathic responses. In the following examples:

   A. Identify which response is most empathic. Explain why.
   B. Why are the other responses nonempathic?
   C. What might be some of the likely consequences of each nonempathic response? How might they interfere with the person's problem-defining and problem-solving efforts?

PERSON: "I let George borrow my French lecture notes last week. Now the test is coming up and he hasn't returned them. I really like George and want to keep his friendship. But how could he be so careless? I want my notes back and am not sure how to get in touch with him. I'm in a real fix."

LISTENER A: "You are irritated with George over his irresponsibility."

LISTENER B: "You could call George's friends and ask them for his phone number."

LISTENER C: "You're frustrated that you can't get your notes before an important test."

LISTENER D: "It's not helpful to get so upset over little things. Let's try taking a few deep breaths to relax."

PERSON: "I wish my boyfriend Henry would stop talking about me to my friends. I know we don't get along in the bedroom. That really worries me. I wonder if we are compatible. But when he talks about it to others, I just want to crawl in a hole and die!"

LISTENER A: "You seem to be very concerned about possible sexual incompatibility."

LISTENER B: "Perhaps now is the time to simply talk with Henry and let him know that you feel his behavior is inappropriate."

LISTENER C: "You know, you and Henry aren't married. Have you considered the possibility that you could avoid a lot of problems by putting sex off until after marriage?"

LISTENER D: "You feel embarrassed when Henry talks about intimate sexual details to friends."

PERSON: "Our family is going on a long vacation in a few weeks. Everyone seems to want to go somewhere different. And all the problems fall on me. I have to get the map, plan the route, buy supplies, and make sure we have enough money."

LISTENER A: "It seems unfair that too many of the duties are falling on you. How does that make you feel?"

LISTENER B: "It's pretty clear to me what's going on with you. If that happened to me, I would be so angry that I would call the whole trip off."

LISTENER C: "These hassles will all blow over once you begin your wonderful trip."

LISTENER D: "Have you checked carefully about the money situation?"

4. When mastering listening skills, Egan suggests starting with the formula response, "You feel _____ because _____." This formula gets you in the habit of looking for content and affect. Later you put your empathic responses in your own language.

In these examples, identify the key feeling and content.

PERSON: "I just found out my father is very sick. In the hospital with heart trouble. He had chest pains, and then trouble breathing. The doctors think it might be a heart attack, but aren't sure. This waiting just drives me up a wall. I'm so rattled I can't sleep."

EXAMPLE LISTENER RESPONSE: "You feel *afraid* because *your father might have had a heart attack*."

PERSON: "I'm a grade school teacher and I never have enough time for myself. I'm always giving tests or grading tests. In addition I teach seven classes a day. I'm constantly preparing lessons between classes. I take several hours of homework home every day, and even have to work in bed and get no sleep. I am just so worn out. So tired. New things come up that I haven't planned for, like having to meet with parents or counsel students. Everything has to be done at once."

LISTENER: "You feel _____ because
_____."

PERSON: "My friend George comes over once a week or
so to visit. We get along real good. He's unemployed, and I often have several days off. Well,
the last few weeks I've been missing things. A
blank video tape. A CD. A few dollars. It's
never anything big. But it's beginning to bother me. I really trust George. And sometimes I
do misplace things."

LISTENER: "You feel _____ because _____."

5. In this exercise, group members generate examples of person problems. Group members generate empathic responses, using the formula "You feel _____ because _____."
6. In the following examples, focus your empathy on people's
attempts to come up with problem definitions or solutions that are
specific, concrete, and realistic.

PERSON: "This is really dumb! We're in this stress group
to talk about things and everyone is so self-
centered. All you can think about is yourself. It
gets me so angry. Sally, I wanted to tell you
that you misunderstood me when I said, 'I'm
at the end of my rope.' But you kept on giving
me advice about what I should do. I couldn't
set you straight."

LISTENER RESPONSE:

PERSON: "When I drive to work I always seem to start a
half hour late. I hit the rush hour at its peak
and arrive in a frantic state of mind. Then I'm
so tense I can't keep my mind on what I'm
doing. I feel really bad that I'm not doing my
best. I wish I could work faster to make up for
lost time. It's funny how such a little thing like
forgetting to set my alarm clock early can mess
up an entire day."

LISTENER RESPONSE:

7. In a group, each person writes down a different empathy script, illustrating a mistake. Assign different types of mistakes to different people so that all mistakes are covered. Collect all scripts and present them to the group. Group members attempt to identify the type of mistake illustrated, and produce a more empathic response. See if you can identify new types of empathy mistakes not discussed in this text.

8. Two group members practice being a listener and other person. The person can either discuss a real problem or one that is made up. The listener attempts to respond with empathy. The group evaluates listener responses, identifying empathy mistakes and skills correctly applied. Use full empathic responses.

9. Before beginning this 2+2 role-playing exercise, person teams meet (apart from listener teams) to select a single member to be the "designated person" and outline the details of a hypothetical problem and possible solutions to discuss. Once problems and designated people have been selected, listener and person teams convene into their four-person groups. The two-person listener team then proceeds to work with the designated person (with the second person of the person team observing and occasionally whispering suggestions to the designated person). Listeners apply empathy to further understand the designated person's problem and attempted solutions.

   At the end of the exercise, the entire group processes the application of empathy. When was it used most effectively? When was it not used? How might the listeners have been more effective?

10. Empathy can facilitate the focusing process as described by Gendlin. How might the various forms of nonempathy discussed in your text interfere with this process?

11. In what ways can empathic listening be a centered activity?

10

Shyness and Social Anxiety

In this chapter we consider shyness and social anxiety. The shy individual lacks the skills to calmly approach, meet, and maintain conversations and contact with others. Someone with social anxiety feels tense in situations where he or she may be observed by others. A key feature of both is that the other person (the one being met, or the observer) need not be a threat or challenge. The shy person is anxious even when the stranger he is meeting is completely unknown, and probably quite harmless. The socially anxious person experiences tension even when she is being observed by complete strangers, or friends. (In chapter 11 we will consider situations in which others are in fact a potential threat or source of anger.)

SECTION 1: CHARACTERISTICS OF SHYNESS AND SOCIAL ANXIETY

Shyness and social anxiety both involve a degree of anxiety. Anxiety is a sense of apprehension and dread over something uncertain that has yet to happen that is not under one's control. Fear is a response to an immediate perceived danger. The fight-or-flight stress arousal response is activated (see chapter 2) to prepare one for emergency action. Panic is an intense fear that occurs when there is no realistic danger, whereas a phobia is an extreme, debilitating, and irrational fear of a specific situation.

Anxiety and fear are normal emotions that are adaptive in many situations. Often they help energize and waken one for effective action. (See Table 10.1 for examples of pathological interpersonal anxiety.) Both emotions are time-limited; on their own, the states of anxiety and fear do not continue, but eventually dissipate. This characteristic is one reason why treatments that involve continued exposure to anxiety and fear-arousing stimuli work.

Shyness and social anxiety have four components: physiological as well as emotional, cognitive, and behavioral. Some physiological symptoms are silent, usually not noted by others: rapidly pounding heart, dizziness,

TABLE 10.1   Interpersonal Anxiety and Psychopathology

Social phobia (social anxiety disorder) and avoidant personality disorders are official mental disorders or psychopathologies listed in the *Diagnostic and Statistical Manual of Mental Disorders,* (DSM-IV-TR; American Psychiatric Association, 2000). A social phobia is "a marked and persistent fear of social or performance situations in which embarrassment may occur." The associated fear must be truly severe and persistent, lasting more than six months and often interfering with life. The key feature of avoidant personality disorder is a "pervasive pattern of social inhibition, feelings of inadequacy, and hypersensitivity to negative evaluation that begins in early adulthood and is present in a variety of contexts." It too must be severe and interfere with life functioning before qualifying as a psychopathology. Although social phobia and avoidant personality disorder share some features with shyness and social anxiety, it should be emphasized that these forms of serious psychopathology must be diagnosed by a qualified mental health professional and require interventions beyond the scope of this book.

nausea, lump in throat, blurred vision, headaches, other aches and pains, chills and "cold hands," tingling fingers, toes, or face, and ringing in the ears. Other symptoms are more public and can be observed by others: shakiness, shortness of breath, blushing, sweatiness, having to go to the bathroom, tearfulness, trembling voice, and nervous laughter. Characteristically, shy and socially anxious individuals often think their symptoms are conspicuous and may contribute to visible interference of performance. In fact, many symptoms are often not noticed.

Shyness and social anxiety can include the emotions of fear and anxiety, as well as possibly sadness and depression. Many of the distorted beliefs associated with lack of assertiveness that we have already considered (chapter 6) also characterize those who are shy and socially anxious. Others (Antony & Swinson, 2000; Bower & Bower, 1991; Curran, Wallander, & Farrell, 1985; Hope, Heimberg, Juster, & Turk, 2000; and Jakubowski & Lange, 1978) speculate that shy and socially anxious individuals are especially likely to be unrealistically perfectionistic and hold themselves to standards they would not apply to others. Often they believe that they are being evaluated by others with equal severity. Shy and socially anxious individuals may be exceptionally self-conscious about their appearance, and unrealistically think others notice and are critical of their weight, hair style, clothing, attractiveness, and so on.

Shy and socially anxious people often display a pattern of anxious avoidant behaviors. Such behaviors may be subtle diversions, such as looking down while talking to others, quickly changing the topic during potentially threatening conversations, or reading a paper while talking to someone. Avoidant behaviors can also be blatant, such as simply refusing to go to a meeting, or escaping early from a party, job interview, or date.

Shy and socially anxious individuals can overprepare for potentially threatening situations. They may bring too many books to class, bring pages of notes to an interview, overdress for a date, and so on. Overall, the behaviors displayed by shy and socially anxious people may actually temporarily reduce anxiety while in the long run contribute to maintaining anxiety. That is, by quickly avoiding or minimizing anxiety, the shy and socially anxious person misses an opportunity to learn to manage anxiety.

In the following two sections we apply the "four pillars" of stress management to shyness and social anxiety. We will examine relaxation, problem-solving, reality-checking, and review/rehearsal strategies. Consistent with the literature on stress management, we will emphasize problem-solving and social skill acquisition when considering shyness and exposure techniques for social anxiety.

SECTION 2: SHYNESS

Relating to and communicating with others is complex. The shy person often feels anxiety and hesitation when thinking about and meeting others, "breaking the ice" and initiating a conversation, maintaining a conversation, ending an encounter, and following up on newly-made friendships. The problem is not so much that the shy person has a pressing issue or want that he or she wants to express; the difficulty is more basic. Shy individuals simply find it difficult communicating about anything. Relaxation and problem-solving can be particularly useful techniques for dealing with this problem.

Relaxation

Different approaches to relaxation have different effects. Some may be more appropriate than others in helping the shy person prepare for a social encounter. Progressive muscle relaxation and autogenic training, because of their tendency to evoke R-State Disengagement when used extensively and alone, may foster withdrawal and interfere with social skills requiring that one approach others. One might become so "tuned out," "laid back," and relaxed, that he or she simply is no longer interested in approaching another person for any reason.

If one's goal is to use relaxation to reduce inhibitions, distance oneself from an immediate problem in order to view it from a new perspective, and enhance brainstorming and divergent thinking, then R-State Disengagement may be desired. Here, progressive muscle relaxation, autogenic training, and perhaps the full array of relaxation techniques might be appropriate.

If one's goal is to increase R-States Energy and Awareness, and possibly positive feelings that may be associated with successful interpersonal encounters (R-State Joy), then yoga stretching and breathing may be appropriate. If relaxation is selected as a reinforcement for successful completion of (and recovery from) a stress management episode, then all techniques are appropriate, especially imagery.

Finally, a personally tailored mini-relaxation is ideal for shyness. Here a brief relaxation exercise is tailor-made for preparing for interpersonal encounters and can be strategically practiced during a stressful encounter. Generally, at the first sign of anxiety, one practices one's mini-relaxation. (See chapter 4.)

Problem-Solving

Getting to know and maintaining relationships with others can be viewed as a problem waiting to be solved. The first step in problem-solving is to clearly and concretely define the problem. Before taking this step, the shy person might have a variety of confusing, vague, and emotional ideas of his or her interpersonal difficulties. For example:

I'm not outgoing enough.
I'm too lonely.
I want people to like me.
I gotta get out more.

Defining a problem involves describing it in concrete and specific terms, actually identifying its "who, what, where, and when." One phrases the problem as a positive "How can I" statement. This typically involves focusing on one concrete incident. For example, an initial definition of the vague problem "I'm not outgoing enough" could be redefined as several concrete specific problems:

How can I find ideas about where to go this Saturday evening to meet people?
How can I meet my neighbor across the hall?
How can I get to know the person I sit next to in temple every Sunday?

Other problem definitions might include expressing opinions about a movie, talking to someone over the phone, inviting friends and strangers over for a party or dinner, or asking someone to spend the night. Remember, in this section we are considering only problems in which there is no potential conflict, problem, or disagreement between oneself and the other person.

Next, one brainstorms possible courses of action and action sequences. For a problem defined as "How can I meet my neighbor across the hall?" one might consider:

Borrowing some cat litter.
Inviting her out for coffee.
Just knocking on her door and introducing oneself.
Waiting for her to go to the laundry room, and then rushing down to do one's own laundry.

Finally, one selects a course of action, considers costs and benefits, and determines a strategy for implementation and reinforcement.

Common Interpersonal Problems and Suggested Strategies

Many useful texts on shyness (including, but not limited to: Antony & Swinson, 2000; Bower & Bower, 1991; Curran, Wallander, & Farrell, 1985; Hope, Heimberg, Juster, & Turk, 2000; and Jakubowski & Lange, 1978) devote considerable space to cataloging various coping strategies one might deploy in various interpersonal situations. These lists are very useful for helping one define a problem and brainstorm solutions. Here are some of the ideas suggested:

Meeting Someone for the First Time

The first step in developing a relationship is getting acquainted. Many people experience anxiety at this stage and harbor a variety of distorted beliefs, such as assuming others will reject them, thinking they will appear foolish, fearing the person will not fit their ideal of what a friend should be, and so on. Once the reality of such beliefs has been checked, there are numerous tactics one could try in developing meeting skills.

An opening line doesn't have to be particularly profound, insightful, or clever. Indeed, openers that appear exceptionally polished can be threatening to others. Simple lines are best. One might want to first think of a set of opening lines. Here are some that researchers have found useful (Kleinke, Meeker, & Staneski, 1986):

"Hi."
"Can you give me directions to _____?"
"Can you help me with _____?"
"Did you see (name a movie or TV show)?"
"Have you read (name an article or book)?"
"I feel a little embarrassed about this, but I'd like to meet you."

"That's a very pretty (sweater, shirt, etc.) you have on."

"You have really nice (hair, eyes, etc.)"

"Since we're both sitting alone, would you care to join me?"

"Is it OK if I sit with you?"

Less effective opening lines include:

"I'm easy. Are you?"

"I've got an offer you can't refuse."

"What's your sign?"

"What is that odor?"

"Didn't we meet in a previous life?"

"Your place or mine?"

"Is that really your hair?"

"You remind me of a woman (man) I used to date."

"Isn't it cold? Let's make some body heat."

As part of the process of developing a set of opening lines, one might consider what makes a good and bad opening line. What should they accomplish? Good opening lines are safe and nonthreatening. They make it easy for the other person to continue, or not continue the conversation. Some are simple, direct, and honest statements. Generally, less effective opening lines:

- Include cute statements
- Involve asking inappropriately intimate or probing questions
- Fill the air with empty talk
- Put oneself or the other person down
- Involve perfunctory ice-breakers and waiting for the other person to jump in and save the conversation.

Questions often make good opening lines, providing they are open-ended and invite more than a simple "yes" or "no." An open-ended question invites the person to share something about themselves, for example:

"That's an interesting book. Could you tell me something about it?"

"What are your thoughts about this cafeteria? I have mixed feelings about it."

In addition to considering possible opening lines, one might consider backup or follow-up lines to say after the other person responds.

One can practice opening lines in a variety of relatively safe settings, including:

- Talking to strangers in waiting lines, bus stops, elevators, etc.
- Asking for directions
- Talk to the cashier in a grocery store.
- Talking to someone sitting next to you in church, a theater, or at a lecture

Following Up an Opening Line and Maintaining a Conversation

Shy people can have difficulty knowing when and how to continue conversations that are already started. They may be afraid of pushing a conversation the other person doesn't want, or nurturing a promising conversation. Here are some hints others have suggested: (Conger & Farrell, 1981; Greenwald, 1977; Kukpke, Calhoun, & Hobbs, 1979):

- Look for signs the other person wants to continue. The best sign is when they give you "free information" about themselves, their thoughts and opinions. Free information goes beyond a simple, perfunctory "yes" and "no." Also, some obvious body signs can tell you if the other person wants to continue. Are they smiling? Facing you? Looking in your direction (or away, at someone else)?
- Pay attention to what the other person is saying. Restate their key points to show you understand and are "with them."
- If the other person expresses a personal feeling, make a point of showing you accept and understand. It can help to empathically restate the feeling.

In maintaining a good conversation, it is important to accurately listen to what others have to say. Any conversation is an exchange of ideas, not a monolog. McKay, Davis, and Fanning (1995) suggest a number of barriers that can interfere with maintaining a conversation (McKay, Davis, & Fanning, 1995):

- Comparing oneself to others. Often one might make negative comparisons with the other person.
- Filtering out certain comments the other person makes. When someone filters, they listen to only certain parts of what is being said. Anxiety and shyness tend to shrink a person's attention span, and the anxious person is more likely to be attentive to cues of liking or rejection. Focus on what the other person is actually saying, and what you think.
- Overrehearsing. Shy and anxious people may spend time practicing in their minds what to say in response. Often the fear is not appearing completely competent. This distorted thought can be countered by recognizing that spontaneous and unpolished replies are often the most endearing.

• Derailing. One might derail a conversation by arbitrarily changing the topic when anxiety makes it boring or tense. Of course, the other person might well conclude that one is not interested.

• Placating and "buttering up" the other person. Shy and anxious people sometimes think they contribute to a conversion by agreeing with everything the other person says. Similarly, they may feel a need to continuously complement the other.

Finally, nonverbal behaviors can contribute to maintaining a conversation. Antony and Swinson (2000) suggest avoiding "closed nonverbal behaviors" that silently suggest one is not interested or is critical. They include:

• Leaning back in a chair
• Sitting or standing far away
• Avoiding eye contact
• Crossing one's arms
• Maintaining a frozen, tense facial expression

In contrast, "open nonverbal behaviors" communicate an interest in the other person and a desire to continue talking:

• Leaning forward while speaking
• Standing a bit closer to others when talking
• Maintaining comfortable eye contact (without staring)
• Keeping arms open, making gestures
• Smiling
• Keeping arms uncrossed

Ending Conversations

Shy and anxious people at times need help in identifying "termination cues," or signs that indicate when a conversation is over or the other person wants to discontinue. There are many strategies for doing this, including (Smith, 1993a):

• Summarizing what you have talked about. ("We seem to agree on who should be president.")
• Simply stating your readiness to leave. ("Well, we've had quite a talk. It is now time for me to go.")
• Showing your interest in the other person. ("I've enjoyed this conversation and would like to meet with you again.")
• Politely excusing yourself. ("I've enjoyed talking with you. I must excuse myself to go home and . . .")
• Stating your plans for what to do next. ("I've planned to do some shopping today. I need to go.")

Maintaining Contact

Shy clients have difficulty not only with initiating contact, but with maintaining relationships that have been newly formed. As a result, potential relationships may cease to grow and even wither away. A number of distorted beliefs can contribute to failure to maintain contact:

- "Let the other person make the first move."
- "I'll call the person later or sometime."
- "If I contact the other person, that will obligate me to more than I am willing to commit to at the moment."
- "If I contact the other person, they will think I'm really hot for them, when that's not exactly how I feel."
- "If I get together with the other person, I might not be sufficiently interesting for them."
- "If we get together, I might find the other person is less interesting that I originally thought, and get bored."
- "If we get together, I might be overwhelmed (or upset) by my strong feelings for the other person."

Just as a shy individual may benefit from brainstorming ways of meeting others, he or she may apply the same strategy to exploring ways of maintaining contact.

Dealing with Rejection

Most negative thoughts people have about making relationships involve the fear of rejection. It can be useful to focus directly on distorted thinking that makes rejection needlessly severe or difficult to deal with. What are some better replacement thoughts? (See chapter 6.)

Exposure, Desensitization, and Stress Inoculation Training

Generally, the key problem with shyness is lack of specific interpersonal skills. When skills are acquired and anxiety prevents carrying them out, then various anxiety-reducing rehearsal strategies may be appropriate. These include simple exposure, desensitization, and stress inoculation training. See chapter 7 for full discussion. We will also consider such anxiety-reducing techniques in the following section.

SECTION 3: SOCIAL ANXIETY

Social anxiety refers to feelings of apprehension one might experience while being observed. Such anxiety can complicate the mastery of basic interpersonal skills we have just considered. For example, when meeting another person for the first time, one might be apprehensive over the possibility that the other person is observing and possibly evaluating one's approach and introduction. When maintaining a conversation, anxiety may be aggravated by an awareness that the other person may notice and be critical of mistakes, awkward gestures and comments, and so on.

However, social anxiety most often appears in performance situations, such as interviews, speaking in public (at meetings, class, church), athletics and public workouts, music and acting, eating with others, and getting married. Anxiety can occur in other nonperformance situations such as using public bathrooms (with others present), writing and filling out forms while others are watching, and shopping in a busy store. Treatment for social anxiety focuses on exposure techniques, including relaxation, problem-solving, and cognitive change strategies.

Relaxation

We have already considered the application of relaxation in interpersonal situations. Many of the same concerns apply here. For example, during an exposure session, do not use techniques that could be conducive to distraction or avoidance (not full 30-minutes sessions of PMR, AT, imagery, meditation); instead use portable energizing techniques such as yoga stretching and imagery. Simple repetition of a relaxation cue ("R - E - L - A - X") may be less likely to evoke Disengagement (perhaps evoking Physical Relaxation, At Ease/Peace, and Energized). For problem-solving and reality-checking, distancing relaxation techniques possibly supplemented by mini-relaxations with PMR, AT, imagery, and meditation are fine. They may foster temporary distancing from the situation so one might objectively consider the problem and reality considerations. Do not use relaxation when problem cues are a person's own physiological or emotional symptoms (Leahy & Holland, 2000); to do so could prematurely reduce anxiety so that it does not have time to habituate.

Reality Checking Specific Beliefs

At the beginning of this chapter, we considered some general distorted beliefs that are associated with anxiety. Once a threatening social situation has been selected, one considers specific distorted beliefs that contribute to anxiety in specific situations. Often, people are fearful of making a fool of themselves, evoking disdain and anger in others, revealing embarrassing or unflattering symptoms, or not being able to control symptoms and feelings. Using the strategies in chapter 6, one checks the reality of distorted thoughts, and identifies realistic replacement thoughts. It can be especially useful to include specific beliefs involving predictions concerning the specific exposure session ("I will be a complete failure," "I will be totally embarrassed," "I will forget everything I am supposed to do.") These can be checked both before and after an exposure session, providing a within-session opportunity for a reality check.

Exposure (or Stress Inoculation Training) Sessions

Social anxiety can be successfully treated with exposure (or stress inoculation training, not considered here). As described in chapter 7, exposure training involves first creating a hierarchy of increasingly threatening exposure situations, all related to a unifying theme (getting closer to the threatening stimulus, more people involved, greater potential for embarrassment, etc.). With imagined (in vitro) exposure, you begin with the least threatening scene and vividly imagine it, using all the senses. Anxiety scores are recorded every few minutes (using the SUDS scale in chapter 7). It is important to include every concrete detail, who, when, what, and where, almost as if replaying a video tape in the mind. Each session should take no more than an hour. Once you can maintain an image without distress (when SUDS scores are about 4), you move on to the next image.

When imagined exposure is practiced with a clinician, he or she narrates the imagery, checking accuracy of details and levels of distress. (At the end of the session, one may reconsider any initial predictions about how the session would go, and rate their accuracy.) Alternatively, a clinician may make a tape of a complete exposure session for clients to play at home several days a week until SUDS scores are reduced.

It is easy to sabotage an exposure session by engaging in distorted unrealistic thinking ("I can't go through with this. This is too much.") It is important to have honestly considered probable lines of distorted thinking ahead of time, and developed honest counters. Cognitive strategies should be applied before, during, and after an exposure session. In other words, no distorted thought should be left unchecked.

It is useful to identify and track avoidant behaviors that might reduce the effectiveness of exposure sessions. Recall that successful exposure requires sustained and intense immersion in an anxiety arousal so that anxiety eventually habituates (which it will if sustained long enough). One learns to "get used" to it by simply putting up with it for a sufficient period of time. However, exposure sessions can be derailed or sabotaged if one avoids and minimizes anxiety in mid-session. Such diversionary maneuvers can include reading, playing a game, listening to the Walkman, nibbling, looking aside, talking about some unrelated topic, and so on. Brainstorming techniques can be used to uncover such diversionary behavior. Using problem-solving, one can then decide on how to minimize the occurrence of diversionary activities (not bringing a book or magazine, leaving the Walkman at home, etc.).

When Casual Exposure Doesn't Work

People often try on their own to reduce social anxiety by directly approaching and getting involved with threatening situations. However, often such informal attempts at exposure fail. Antony and Swinson (2000) caution that one cause for failure is that everyday exposure situations are often unpredictable and uncontrollable. One might be asked unexpectedly to speak in front of others, introduce oneself, and so on. Perhaps the most important key to reducing the potential threat of a situation is to render it as predictable and controllable as possible. Systematic exposure sessions, when done realistically, are ideal ways of achieving this.

In addition, casual informal attempts at exposure are often too brief or infrequent to work. A person might try shopping in a crowded store, experience social anxiety, and quickly leave. This avoidance derails the exposure process, preventing a sustained period of anxiety (which spontaneously dissipates in time). In fact, by quitting early, the person actually reinforces and strengthens avoidance and the distorted thinking that he or she can't cope with the anxiety-arousing situation. Similarly, people may entertain subtle ways of avoiding a situation that minimize sustained anxiety (drinking, taking drugs, taking someone along, hiding in a corner, reading).

Everyday Exposure Opportunities

Many mild forms of social anxiety can be treated by using safe everyday opportunities (Antony & Swinson, 2000: Bower & Bower, 1991; Hope, Heimberg, Juster, & Turk, 2000). Here, one deliberately brainstorms and selects situations that might likely evoke interpersonal anxiety. One then deliberately seeks out one or two such situations. For example, a clinician might suggest to a client the following:

- Job interviews. Apply for a few jobs you are not particularly interested in (safe interviews with no consequence to you). Call up job contacts for work posted in the paper, inquire about the job, and make a case that you might be right for the job.
- Speaking to authority figures. At church or temple, ask to talk with the priest, minister, rabbi, etc. about the sermon. Ask to talk to the manager of a store about a problem you have had with service (or an item). Call the cable company and request to talk to a supervisor about your lousy service. Find the most distinguished looking older person waiting for the bus, and ask them to give directions.
- Requesting information, help. Walk up to every 10th total stranger in the street and ask for directions. Ask the student sitting next to you to explain a point.

- Expressing opinions in public. When with friends, make a point of expressing and explaining your opinion during a discussion.
- Public speaking. Decide ahead of time to make a point at a meeting. Ask a relatively extended question in class in front of others.
- Eating in front of others. Eat in a fast-food restaurant rather than at home. Eat with chopsticks (at Asian restaurants only). Go to crowded restaurants.
- Writing in front of others. Write a check rather than pay in cash. Go to banks and stores when they are busy. Volunteer to take minutes, or chalkboard notes, during a meeting.
- Fear of making mistakes. Try a new hobby or sport (one in which you a re likely to make a mistake) in public. Make a harmless mistake on purpose. Play games you are bad at. Deliberately spill water at a table.

EXERCISES

1. Over the week, go to a setting where others typically meet each other for the first time (church, cafeteria, tavern, health club). Listen to conversations. What are some of the effective and ineffective introductions and follow-up discussions you observe?
2. What are the best strategies you have for continuing a discussion with someone new?
3. Role-play a situation in which you experience anxiety when approaching others. First, incorporate what you would ordinarily do and say. Then repeat the role-play exercise, incorporating revisions you have thought of or that have been suggested by your trainer or (in a group) by others.
4. Role-play a situation in which you experience anxiety maintaining a conversation. (Use instructions in Exercise 3.)
5. In what situations are you most likely to experience social anxiety?
6. What are your cues for the social anxiety situation just listed?
7. Construct a hierarchy of 10 social anxiety scenes for the situation you listed.
8. What distorted beliefs contribute to social anxiety in this situation?
9. In what ways can dealing with shyness and social anxiety be centered activities?

11

Conflict, Anger, and Aggression

Conflict, anger, and aggression are a part of life, and a major part of stress. How can one productively express negative thoughts and feelings that may provoke disagreement or hostility? What are useful ways of making challenging requests, disagreeing, and expressing feelings of anger? How does one deal with anger and aggression from others? Although conflict, anger, and aggression are often not pleasant, they can have healthy consequences. They can provide needed energy and motivation to change. They can sensitize one to problems that may be hidden. Conflict, anger, and aggression are destructive when they are irrational (as with prejudice, bigotry, and homophobia). They can contribute to physical pathology if not realistically dealt with; indeed the chronic overexpression of anger can be just as personally destructive as holding anger in.

SECTION 1: NEGATIVE ASSERTIONS OR REQUESTS THAT MIGHT BE CHALLENGED (OR LEAD TO CONFLICT)

Many assertions and requests are very unlikely to lead to potential conflict. Innocuous self-disclosures ("I'm a little hungry."), inquiries ("Do you have the time?"), or positive invitations ("May I buy you a drink?") may create stress when one is shy or socially anxious (chapter 10). However, sometimes assertions and requests may challenge or threaten others, and even (in extreme cases) lead to conflict. Consider the following example in which Chuck has invited his friend Buck to a party:

CHUCK: "We've been at this party for 2 hours. Where is everyone?"

BUCK: "I'm bored. What a stupid waste!"

CHUCK: "Well, I'm sorry I invited you. I'm hurt."

Clearly Chuck was angered by Buck's negative assertion. Simple but potentially threatening negative assertions are less likely to be provocative when they are presented objectively (noting the "4 W's"—Who, What, When, Where), meet the reality-checking criteria of chapter 6, and include an empathic understanding of the other person:

CHUCK: "We've been at this party for 2 hours. Where is everyone?"

BUCK: "I agree. Two hours is a long time. You seem a little tired. I'm bored."

CHUCK: "Yeah. Let's go to the pub."

Often when one makes a request from another person, there is the potential the request may be denied or viewed as a threat. This is particularly true if one is requesting a behavior change ("Please don't talk so loud in the theater"). Bower and Bower's (1991) DESC script provides a useful and structured four-step format for behavior-change requests:

D - DESCRIBE: Clearly and objectively state the other person's behavior or words that are a problem.
CORRECT EXAMPLE: "Yesterday you stated you would meet me at the mall at noon so we could eat. I arrived at the mall, and you were not there."
INCORRECT EXAMPLE: "Why are you so careless? You never seem to follow through."

E - EXPRESS: State your thoughts and feelings in reaction to the described behavior.
CORRECT EXAMPLE: "I felt confused, and then a little irritated."
INCORRECT EXAMPLE: "I'm just fed up with your stupidity."

S - SPECIFY: Present a specific request of the other person.
CORRECT EXAMPLE: "The next time we arrange for lunch, and you cannot make it, please call me ahead of time."
INCORRECT EXAMPLE: "It would be good if you could be more considerate of others."

C - CONSEQUENCES: Outline the positive consequences for oneself and the other person if the request is followed.
CORRECT EXAMPLE: "I will feel better about having lunch with you and won't have to worry about whether or not you will show up."
INCORRECT EXAMPLE: "If you don't straighten up, things will just get worse."

Bower and Bower provide some useful guidelines for each stage:

DESCRIBE

Describe behavior, not your own feelings. Use concrete terms, stating who, when, what, and where. Don't guess at the other person's reasons.

EXPRESS

Calmly state your own feelings, relating them to the specific behavior, not the whole person.

SPECIFY

Ask for realistic concrete, behavioral change, indicating again who, what, when, and where. Acknowledge the other person's wants.

CONSEQUENCES

Be honest, realistic, concrete, and explicit. Don't bribe or threaten.

It can be useful to rehearse one's DESC script, possibly after practicing relaxation.

SECTION 2: DEALING WITH ONE'S OWN ANGER

Some people have difficulty expressing feelings of anger in a useful way. They may argue, explode with rage, or even verbally attack. In dealing with one's own anger, we begin with a consideration of cues that can indicate the onset of anger and aggressive behavior, and the need for some type of aggression management. The first cues include provocative cognitions, the most common of which include the belief or perception that (Goldstein & Keller, 1987):

- Someone else has, or is about to violate your expectations of what is right and expected
- Someone else has, or is about to insult, hurt, or provoke another person significant to you
- Someone else has, or is about to insult, hurt, or provoke you
- You have encountered a serious frustration to achieving your goals
- You have encountered an appropriate target for expressing irrational/habitual or religion-based feelings of prejudice, bigotry, homophobia, or dislike

Emotional and physiological cues of anger are often the most visible signs of an impending aggressive outburst for an impulsive person. Emotional cues include, of course, feelings of anger, hostility, irritation, frustration, rage, and so on. At times the aggressive person may confuse anxiety and fear with anger, and will need assistance (through empathic listening) to articulate. Physiological cues of anger arousal include those related to striated (voluntary) muscle tension (making a fist, raising one's shoulders, puffing up one's chest, tightening one's muscles, standing tall, frowning, furrowing one's brow, clenching and grinding one's teeth, squinting, etc.). Some cues are autonomic cues (flushed cheeks, rapid heart beat, rapid shallow breathing, stomach difficulties). Behavioral cues of an impending anger attack might include preparations to attack (rolling up one's sleeves and making a fist, reaching for the phone to make an aggressive phone call, or walking towards the offending other person).

Early Anger Management Strategies (Catching it in the Bud)

Once one has identified cues of impending aggression, one can consider anger management strategies. If possible, it is desirable to deal with problems early, before they snowball into more complex crises. Typically, early strategies involve cooling off and checking the reality of angry thoughts.

Relaxation

Relaxation can be an effective early anger-reducer to be applied at the moment one detects an anger cue. If a client has developed a mini-relaxation targeted to anger (chapter 4), it may be used. If a mini-relaxation is not available, little time is available, and the situation involves others, I recommend the passive breathing exercises discussed in chapter 4. These include *inhaling through nose, exhaling through lips,* taking *occasional deep breaths,* and *focused breathing.* Of these, research suggests that taking occasional deep breaths may be the most effective (Smith & Jackson, 2001). The instructions are:

> Let yourself breathe easily and naturally. When you are ready, take in a full deep breath, filling your lungs and abdomen with good, refreshing air. Pause. And when you are ready, relax. And slowly let the air flow out, very smoothly and gently. And now, just continue breathing normally for a while.

In addition, strategies fostering Disengagement and Physical Relaxation may be particularly useful for helping a client "pull away" from anger. Most effective might be PMR and AT. The "tense up - let go" cycles of PMR can be particularly appealing for angry individuals. "Tensing up" during a PMR session can be presented as something like the angry clenching (making a fist and tightening up one's arms and legs for a fight, furrowing one's brow) for an angry confrontation, and "letting go" like the release of needless anger. For more skilled relaxation practitioners, imagery and meditation may be appropriate.

Reality Checking

Much anger is the result of unrealistic expectations, distorted perceptions, or failure to consider all the possible causes of a problem. Simply pausing, and taking time to consider all aspects of a provocative situation, can be enough to reduce the potential for anger. All of the forms of distorted thinking considered in chapter 6 can be potential sources of distorted personal anger, including;

Fortune-telling. "Whatever you do, you'll end up attacking me."

Unrealistic Isolation. "I just don't belong. Since everyone's out for themselves, out to get me, I'll just be by myself."

Needless Perfectionism. "They're always looking at me with hostility because I don't live up to high enough standards."

Childlike Fantasy. "Things should go my way; it really angers me when they don't."

Helplessness. "I can't solve any of this by myself. It makes me angry that others won't always help me out."

Novaco's Anger Management Stress Inoculation Program

Novaco (1975) has offered an approach to managing anger that is essentially similar to stress inoculation training; elements are central to many contemporary approaches (Deffenbacher, 1999). He suggests breaking a potential anger problem-situation into four stages, each with its own coping goals and strategies (Note the similarities to our phases of stress in chapter 7). First, a client considers which stage is a problem. Then, he or she brainstorms and evaluates coping strategies. Here is a modification of Novaco's approach, with some of his more useful illustrations:

1. *Preparing for provocation (pre-stress).* If a client can anticipate a confrontation that has potential for creating conflict and anger, he or she can prepare ahead of time. Preparations can include *active coping* plans ("Let me plan what I will do," "I will make sure my friends are around that day in case I need to talk with them," "I might get upset, but there is no need for violence"), *checking the reality* of thoughts to defuse conflict or aggression ("I should remember not to take things too seriously," "This will be a good chance to see if I remember to keep my cool," "At least I will be able to practice my coping skills"), and *relaxation and defensive strategies* to reduce or avoid tension ("I know how to handle my anger," "If I get overwhelmed with anger, I'll do my relaxation," "I'm still a good person, even if things go wrong," "Just keep a good sense of humor").

2. *Impact and confrontation (onset-stress).* In the next phase, the incident is just beginning. The confrontation has occurred. Once again, a client can plan active coping strategies ("Just talk things through," "Take one moment at a time," "Don't try to put him/her down, just focus on the facts," "Just roll with the punches," "I'm not going to let the other person push my anger

buttons," "Look for the positive and don't jump to negative conclusions"), reality checking ("I'm in control," "I know what to do," "For someone to be as angry as him/her, they must have real problems coping"), or relaxation and defensive strategies ("Stay cool and relax," "What the other person says about me doesn't really matter in the long run," "The person who wins is the one who knows how to learn from mistakes").

3. *Coping with arousal (mid-stress).* In the midst of a confrontation, a client runs the risk of unexpected and disruptive increments in arousal. These can be anticipated and managed through active coping ("I'll let him/her continue screaming and yelling and stand back while he/she wastes his/her time, and looks like a fool," "Whoa, let's slow down, and take the problem point by point," "Let's try to reason and treat him/her with respect," "I'll ignore the crazy accusations and just focus constructively on the facts"), reality checking ("Getting more and more tense doesn't help one bit," "I have every right to be annoyed, but let's keep things in perspective," "I know how to cope"), and relaxation and defense ("Take ten deep breaths," "I'm going to ask for a five minute time off period," "I've had enough and am going to forget about the problem until I have a calm, clear head").

4. *Reflecting on the provocation (post-stress).* Finally, when the confrontation is over stress can still continue. Here it is useful to anticipate two general outcomes: what to do when the conflict is unresolved ("Just forget it," "At least I can learn from my mistakes," "Let's look at this in perspective," "OK, relax") or resolved successfully ("I did pretty well," It could have been much worse," "I think I learned something").

SECTION 3: DEALING WITH AGGRESSION AND HOSTILITY FROM OTHERS

Novaco's four stages may not be enough to deal with an angry confrontation, especially if the other person is consumed and blinded by rage. Here the objectives and strategies may be a bit different.

Direct Aggression

Establishing an Environment not Conducive to Destructive Conflict

Often it is useful simply to calm the other person down. Goldstein and Keller (1987) offer some very useful advice for relaxing a potentially hostile or aggressive person and establishing an atmosphere not conducive to destructive conflict. I have somewhat revised and added to their suggestions one might give a client:

CHANGE THE SETTING

If possible, move one's encounter to a setting where anger cues and reinforcements (such as a potential audience, arousing stimuli, or reminders of whatever transgression may have occurred) are not present, and cues suggestive of calm (and mature problem-solving, if possible) are present. For example, if you accidentally bumped someone walking past you in the crowded park (spilling a drink on their coat), and they turn to you ready to argue, suggest taking the discussion to a quiet spot off the sidewalk.

MODEL CALMNESS

Simply be and look relaxed, not only in voice tone and content, but in body language. Smith (1999b) has identified three general types of relaxed behavior: breathing (slow breathing pace, even breathing rhythm, greater use of diaphragmatic "stomach" breathing, and reduced chest extension during breathing); posture (shoulders relaxed and slightly sloped, palms, arms, and legs slightly open and not clenched or closed); and muscle activity (no nervous movements, chewing, fidgeting, blinking).

ENCOURAGE RATIONAL AND PROBLEM-SOLVING TALK

It can be useful to ask the other person to discuss what they might constructively do about the problem, rather than ask the person to explain why they are angry (a tactic which can actually increase anger). One should ask the aggressive person to speak slowly, more quietly, and simply so they can be understood better.

LISTEN EMPATHICALLY

Using the suggestions in chapter 9, begin by paraphrasing what the other person is saying. Make it clear you are interested and listening. At least restate or rephrase their comments. If possible, focus on problem-solving empathy.

REWARD CALM BEHAVIOR

When the other person displays reduction in distracting anger or aggression, gently praise them, taking care not to be condescending or patronizing. "I appreciate your frankness and openness; it helps me understand where you are coming from; I think we are more likely to work things out." In rewarding such behavior, reassure the other person that you believe a nonaggressive approach can be very helpful in solving problems.

Goals for Dealing with Aggressive Behavior

The first goal of dealing with aggressive and manipulative behavior is to conduct a reality check and determine if the aggression or manipulation is real or imagined. Next, one conducts simple problem-solving (suggested by Jakubowski & Lange, 1978). In sum, we can consider four overall goals in dealing with aggressive behavior of others:

- Do a reality check on whether aggression is real or imagined.
- Get to the source of the problem.
- Accomplish your goals.
- Limit the other person's aggressive behavior, possibly help them meet their goals.

DO A REALITY CHECK ON WHETHER AGGRESSION IS REAL OR IMAGINED

Consider the discussion earlier on checking one's own anger. Is the perceived aggression of another person real or imagined? What information is necessary in order to make that determination? What questions should be asked?

GET TO THE SOURCE OF THE PROBLEM

- Temporarily ignore the hostile content of someone's remark, and empathically observe the distress. Examples:

  OTHER PERSON: "I can't stand it when you keep on acting like that I just don't know what to do. I'm completely fed up."

  ONESELF: "I sense your frustration and irritation."

  OTHER PERSON: "You promised to take me out last week and didn't do a thing. You must take me for granted. I really feel like I've been put down."

  ONESELF: "Yes, I can see you're pissed off I didn't remember your birthday."

- Ask for a clarification. When an angry person confuses an issue with emotion, or adds irrelevant issues, acknowledge or ignore the emotional content ("I know you are angry about this. But it is not clear to me just what I did wrong.") and focus on the apparent problem.
- Focus on the issue. Use the concrete, specific, and realistic problem-defining strategies of this text and ask for one specific illustration of a concrete and specific problem behavior. Which goal was not being met?
- Tell the other person the message you hear. The other person can then adjust and present their complaint in a more useful way.

  ONESELF: You have explained how I am an insensitive, crass, careless pig who can't get anything right. That puts me in a place where I have no idea what I can do to make things better.

  OTHER PERSON: "Well, I guess I was going overboard. It's your clumsiness that gets to me."

ONESELF: "I'm clumsy. That's awfully vague. I still don't know where to figure that out. Do I make mistakes at work, home, with children, while driving? Help me out."

OTHER PERSON: "No, no. This is it. Yesterday you promised to finish my report. You did, but left out two important paragraphs I had in the original. I had to retype the entire project. I felt irritated."

- Get the other person to rephrase their problem in terms that are concrete, specific, and realistic.

ACCOMPLISH YOUR GOAL

Another strategy is for the person to focus on what they want out of an aggressive encounter. Here are a number of techniques Jakubowski and Lange suggest:

- Ignore the other person's aggressive comments and simply persist with what you want to say.
- Simply and directly dismiss the relevance of what the other person is saying, and return to your main point.
- Put the aggression aside as an issue that can be dealt with later; return to your goal.

LIMIT THE EFFECTS OF AGGRESSION

Sometimes, the main problem is to limit aggressive behavior that is going nowhere or escalating to dangerous proportions. Again, here are some suggestions:

- Ask questions to prompt awareness of the aggressive behavior.
- Behave in a calm, problem-solving manner, in direct contrast to the aggressive behavior being displayed.
- Provide direct and specific negative feedback.
- Treat a putdown as a neutral comment (ignore the emotional component, and focus on what might be true).
- Sort out fact from judgement and interpretation. Focus on the facts.
- Announce the intent to escalate your assertions, and wish for a contract to end the aggression.

APPLY THE DESC SCRIPT

The Bower and Bower's (1991) DESC script has considerable potential for dealing with provocations from others. Here one first describes the concrete specifics of the provocation, expresses one's feelings in response, specifies a concrete behavior change request, and outlines the positive consequences if a solution can be found.

Suggest Negotiation

Once another person's anger has subsided, and disagreement persists, it may be appropriate to offer an invitation to engage in some sort of negotiation in an attempt to resolve issues in a mutually acceptable fashion. See later section.

Complex Aggression

Dealing with Unproductive Hostile, Manipulative, and Passive-Aggressive Behavior

A special type of interpersonal problem emerges when others interfere with one's attempts to solve problems realistically and assertively. Subtle forms of unproductive hostile, manipulative, and passive-aggressive behavior are often disguised and may even appear innocent on the surface. One step in coping with such behaviors is to recognize their cues and consequences, especially costs and benefits to oneself and the other person. Several self-help books provide useful catalogs of suggestions (Alberti & Emmons, 1982; Bower and Bower, 1976; McMullin, 1986), some of which can be usefully offered to clients as suggestions:

ARGUING NEEDLESSLY

Others can avoid problems by arguing about a relatively minor or unimportant topic. Examples:

> "You're asking why I didn't call last night. Well, since when do I have to always be by a phone?"

> "You think I am having relations with another woman. Well, just what do you mean by 'relations'?"

> "I recognize I promised to do some weekend work at the office. But isn't Friday afternoon really considered 'weekend' by most people?"
> • Possible payoff to other person: They control the direction of the discussion.
> • Possible cost to oneself: Derailed from making or considering one's topic.

BLAMING

Another person blames someone or something else for the problem one has brought up, thereby creating a distraction. Examples:

> "Well, it's your fault I didn't come to pick you up for work. You should always call me twice to remind me. You know that."

"Please recognize how difficult it is for me to avoid expressing my anger physically. My parents brought me up to be a very physical person."

"I'll be more than happy to pay more attention to you. Once you start acting decent."

- Possible payoff to other person: They get off the hook and don't have to accept responsibility for their actions.
- Possible cost to oneself: One might begin to blame oneself.

BLANKET DENIAL

The other person simply does not accept one's challenge, and effectively terminates the discussion. Examples:

"I never said I would do the dishes."

"Your worries are just in your head and have no substance."

"This is a nonissue. Why are we even considering it?"

- Possible payoff to other person: Discussion is terminated. The denier puts him or herself in the dominant role as the final arbiter.
- Possible cost to oneself: One might feel one's point reflected distorted thinking, such as catastrophizing.

DISCOUNTING

Discounting is similar to blanket denial, except one simply reduces the significance or importance of the topic. Examples:

"Come on, go easy on me!"

"Why is this such a problem for you? We can work this out, it's such a little deal."

"You've made a mountain out of a molehill."

- Possible payoff to other person: Similar to blanket denial. The other person can come across as mature and calm.
- Possible cost to oneself: One wonders if he or she is getting too emotional.

DISTRACTION

The other person prevents one from assertively making their point or defining a problem with irrelevant statements. Examples:

"Oh, what kind of aftershave is that?"

"You're so sexy when you're frustrated."

"Gee, you're getting pushy."

- Possible payoff to other person: They prevent one from talking about what one wants to talk about. Confuse or upset person.
- Possible cost to oneself: One does not get to finish what he or she was planning to say or do. Feels hurt, put down, or ignored.

JOKING

The other person uses humor to try to defuse a situation. Examples:

"You questioned why I am sometimes late. Well, how else can I be sure that you are paying attention?"

"Why did I break my promise to mow the lawn? I just wanted it to grow more so I could have even more fun mowing it next time."

"I know you don't like it when I yell at you in public. But it sure helps build my singing voice!"

- Possible payoff to the other person: They assume a role that is "above" the conflict.
- Possible cost to oneself: One feels demeaned, and wonders if one's point was exaggerated.

PSYCHOLOGIZING

The other person tries to divert attention by offering psychological-sounding explanations for one's behavior that focus on childhood history, family problems, and hidden motives. Examples:

"You women are always that way."

"You sure are getting defensive all of a sudden."

"You must have problems with intimacy with members of the opposite gender; otherwise, you would go home with me."

- Possible payoff to other person: One assumes a controlling role as "expert" (psychologist).
- Possible cost to oneself: Because most psychological accusations are unprovable, one can become diverted and preoccupied with considering the accusation.

SILENT TREATMENT

The other person simply ignores you or refuses to communicate.

- Possible payoff to other person: Conflict avoided.
- Possible cost to oneself: One has no idea what is causing the silent treatment, leading to diverting confusion.

VICTIMIZATION

The other person plays the role of the victim, and pretends to be violated, hurt, insulted, or helpless.

> "You know I'm sensitive about work. So why do you keep asking me why I'm late?"

> "I've been dealing with some personal problems lately, and just haven't been dealing with others well."

> "Your accusations could not have come at a worse time. Anything that could have gone wrong has."

- Possible payoff to other person: Distracting play for sympathy.
- Possible cost to oneself: One may simply give up one's assertive point out of guilt and compassion.

YES . . . YES . . . YES

The other person profusely and repeatedly agrees one's point, often offering frequent apologies.

> "You are so right and I am so wrong. I am very, very sorry. I feel so guilty about what I have done. How could I have been so stupid? I'm so, so sorry."

> "Yes, you don't have to say anything more. I know exactly what you are saying and, you know, you are right. I agree with you totally. End of discussion."

> "I've already agreed that I am completely and totally responsible. There really isn't anything else to talk about. Let me buy you a coffee."

- Possible payoff to other person: A play for sympathy. By filling the air with talk, one is prevented from continuing.
- Possible cost to oneself: One may feel guilty.

In sum, when another person does not treat one as a peer or equal, or seems to want to dominate, manipulate, hurt, or attack, they are behaving aggressively. Goals include, again, pointing out and stopping the verbal aggression, and focusing on productive problem-solving. Often DESC scripts are particularly useful.

Dealing With Hate and Potential Violence (Prejudice, Bigotry, Racism, Homophobia, etc.)

Many of the techniques and strategies we have considered can apply to situations in which a client is the recipient of hostility based on prejudice, bigotry, racism, homophobia, and irrational dislike (dislike for women, thin people, older people, people with glasses, students, non-Christians, redheads, etc.). However, often when such irrational hatred is expressed there may well be no underlying problem to solve. To pursue a problem-solving agenda may well aggravate hostility ("How dare you, a member of _____ detestable subgroup, suggest a solution.") When problem-solving seems out of the picture, one needs to clearly define the problem, what one wants to accomplish. Five possible goals include:

- Exit the encounter as safely and quickly as possible
- Defuse the potential for escalating aggression
- Assertively express one's thoughts and feelings about the encounter
- Educate the perpetrator, assuming this person is not violent and he or she is open to edification
- Make an educational/social/political/spiritual point for the benefit of others who may be present

SECTION 4: NEGOTIATION

What happens when two assertive people have equally reasonable requests? Negotiation is the process of applying simple problem-solving to a problem two individuals have. It can be useful to begin with relaxation, and then consider any distorted thoughts that might interfere with the process of give and take. Such thoughts might include:

There must always be a winner or a loser.
If I don't get what I want, I've failed.
This is a contest of strength, with the strongest person winning.
Disagreement should always be avoided.
There is only one way of resolving it, the one that I have already thought of.
Someone's going to get hurt.

Such negative thinking needs to be approached with more realistic and adaptive thoughts, starting with overall goals. In negotiation, two peers take on a win-win or compromise strategy, recognizing that with honest communication, both parties may well achieve their goals, or both may have to give a little in order to get what they want.

Psychologist Arnold Goldstein has offered much useful advice on negotiation (Goldstein & Keller, 1987). The first thing he recommends to keep in mind is that effective negotiations don't just happen. He suggests one think out one's position ahead of time, pick a neutral (and private setting) and negotiate in person.

Others have suggested various steps in the negotiation process (Jakubowski & Lange, 1978; Goldstein & Keller, 1987). Generally, they involve clearly stating one's own position, listening to and checking one's understanding of the other person's position, and, once it is clear both parties clearly understand each other, proposing a compromise.

When Nothing Works: The Final DESC Script

Some differences simply cannot be reconciled and both parties may have to settle with accepting no resolution. Here, a reasonable goal can be to assertively express oneself, rethink one's goals, and go on living. One might choose to terminate an unsuccessful negotiation with a clear and concise summary of what has transpired, focusing on both one's own wants, thoughts, feelings, and behavior as well as those of the other person. Again, a DESC script can be a useful tool, with the DESCRIBE line focusing on the failed negotiation process:

DESCRIBE (SUMMARIZES BOTH POSITIONS): "We have negotiated this problem for three days. Both of us have made a reasonable attempt to offer solutions and compromises. But we still haven't reached a solution."

EXPRESS: "I feel very frustrated when I can't negotiate a solution. But I also feel resigned that perhaps that is how it will have to be."

SPECIFY: "Let me suggest that we stop our negotiations and accept that we both have legitimate, but irreconcilable, differences."

CONSEQUENCES: "I would like to leave at least feeling that we made our best effort to resolve our differences, and that we still respect each other."

EXERCISES

1. Throughout the week, look for others engaged in conflict. Note any attempts by one person to relax the other person. Describe the situation, what was done, and what could have been done.

2. Recall an angry conflict situation you have experienced. What attempts were made to relax the other person? What could have been done?

3. Think of a plausible angry encounter you might have in the future (or use one you have had in the past). Write a detailed script for the situation, incorporating Novaco's four stages. Include what you would do.

4. Role-play an angry encounter. In a class or group setting, the recipient of anger leaves the room. The designated provoking person consults with others in the group as to what behaviors he or she will display. When the recipient returns, role-play an angry encounter, with the recipient attempting to relax the provoking person. The group observes and notes what was attempted, what worked, and what did not work.

5. Throughout the week, look for manipulative and insensitive behavior others have displayed. What type of behavior was it, according to the text? What were the cues and possible costs? How might one have dealt with the provocative behavior?

6. Recall or think of a likely conflict situation. Script out how you might achieve the four goals suggested by Jakubowski and Lange:

   - Do a reality check on whether aggression is real or imagined
   - Get to the source of the problem.
   - Accomplish your goals.
   - Limit the other person's aggressive behavior, possibly help them meet their goals.

7. Role-play a conflict situation. First select a situation. In a group, first discuss the details of the situation. Then brainstorm what could specifically be said to achieve appropriate goals. Then have two people act out the situation, applying the goals they remember. Discuss which were successfully applied and which could be applied.

8. Write a DESC script for a conflict situation. Group members (or a trainer) evaluate each step according to the criteria in the book.

9. What cognitive distortions do you most associate with problems with anger? What are effective counter statements for each?

10. In what ways can dealing with aggression and conflict be centered activities?

Part IV

Task Completion Skills: Time Management, Procrastination, and Positive Beliefs

12

Time Management

One of the first problems people have in applying stress management techniques is finding time to practice. Whether the task is practicing a relaxation technique, reading a chapter, or doing a homework exercise, no technique or strategy in this book can work unless one makes time to explore and apply. Time management is not only a stress management topic, but it is a prerequisite for all other approaches to stress management to work.

People often think of time as a source of stress and complain about not having enough of it or being pressured by it. However, it is misleading to think of time as a stress stimulus; no strategy can alter the fact that there are only 24 hours in a day. When people have concerns about time, they usually have problems with too much work, not enough recreation, conflicts between equally unpleasant (or pleasant) tasks, missed deadlines, feeling overwhelmed by trivia, inability to do what they want because of unfinished tasks, and so on.

SECTION 1: THE GREAT MYTH OF MULTITASKING (AND OTHER DISTORTED BELIEFS)

Perhaps the most common distorted belief concerning time management is the notion that doing several tasks at once, *multitasking*, saves time. It is tempting to think that simultaneously writing a report, answering the phone, and filling out an accounting inventory might enable one to complete these three tasks in, say, one third the time. Indeed, some popular psychologists have praised the claimed capacity of the human brain to do many things (note the frequent erroneous observation that people use only "10 percent of their brains").

In fact, multitasking appears to waste time. Individuals who do several tasks at once must frequently switch from one task to another. One almost never actually completes several tasks at the same time, as a pianist might play a bass melody with the left hand while simultaneously playing a main melody with the right. Rubinstein, Meyer, and Evans (2001) have noted that shifting from task to task involves two unconscious and time-consuming activities: goal-shifting ("I want to do this now instead of that") and rule activation ("I'm turning off the rules for doing that and turning on the rules for doing this").

Consider the tasks of surfing the Web and proofreading a report for errors. The rules for surfing include using the mouse to move the cursor, double clicking screen choices, clicking the "back" key to return to a previous screen, pushing another button once to bookmark a page, and so on. The rules for proofreading are different and might include first skimming a page for obvious mistakes, reading the report one word at a time to check for spelling, and then rereading the report paragraph by paragraph to see if one's points are clear. Someone who surfs and proofreads simultaneously actually is switching from one task to another. The decision that it is time to stop, say, proofreading and begin surfing takes a fraction of a second. And then, the decision to "get in the mind-set" of surfing, and bring to mind how one surfs takes another fraction of a section. Although each switch may waste only a second or so, the multitasker makes many switches, wasting much time. What is more efficient? Prioritizing and organizing one's time.

In my experience other cognitive distortions associated with problems with time management (as well as procrastination) often include: Fortune-Telling, Minimizing, Childhood Fantasy, and Helplessness. For example, different clients having difficulty with procrastination and time management might think:

"My plans to get a new job are going to fail. So why try?"

"People say I should plan ahead what courses I will take next semester. It's not that important."

"Managing time is a stupid, compulsive thing to do. Only nerds do this sort of thing."

"Why plan? Everything will turn out fine."

"Why plan? My actions won't make any difference anyway."

I suggest the reader consult chapter 6 and creatively consider other ways each of these might contribute to problems with time management and procrastination.

Alan Lakein (1973) and Harold Greenwald (1973) have offered useful time management ideas that are frequently cited in the literature. Their suggestions can be organized into four categories, generally supported by research (Macan, 1994). (Often these are presented as sequential steps, although I find each can be productively completed by itself.)

SECTION 2: THE TIME INVENTORY

Most people have a vague idea of how they spend time throughout the day. Often taking inventory can reveal wasteful activities and motivate one to change. To do this, one might first divide the day into half-hour segments and record typical activities for each. Here is how a college freshman outlined her activities:

Daily log

8:30–9:00	Start breakfast
9:00–9:30	Eat breakfast
9:30–10:00	Watch TV
10:00–10:30	Study by self
10:30–11:00	Class
11:00–12:00	Class
12:00–12:30	Go for walk
12:30–1:00	Watch TV
1:00–1:30	Lunch
1:30–2:00	Watch TV
2:00–2:30	Walk
2:30–3:00	Snacks
3:00–3:30	Watch TV
3:30–4:00	Talk to friends
4:00–4:30	Walk home
4:30–5:00	Watch TV
5:00–5:30	Study by self
5:30–6:00	Do homework with friends
6:00–7:00	Dinner
7:00–8:00	Talk with parents
8:00–9:00	Watch TV
9:00–10:00	Get ready for bed
10:00–10:30	Study
10:30–11:00	Talk with friends
11:00–11:30	Talk with friends

Such an initial log is the beginning raw material of time management. By itself it is not particularly informative and can be confusing. The first step in finding order in what might seem to be a disordered list is to identify the categories of activities one does. Our student identified the following:

Types of activities
Studying
In class
Eating and preparing for eating

Socializing
Getting ready for bed, dressing, etc.
Travel
TV

Next, one divides the day into three segments, perhaps morning to 12 noon; 12 noon to 6 P.M.; 6 P.M. to bedtime. Using the above list of types of activities, one indicates how many hours are spent on each for each time period.

Types of activities done in morning, afternoon, and evening
  Morning to 12 noon
    Studying . . . . 30 min
    In class . . . . 1 hr
    Eating and preparing for eating . . . . 1 hr
    Socializing 0
    Getting ready for bed, dressing, etc. . . . . 30 min
    Travel 0
    TV 1
  12 noon to 6 P.M.
    Studying . . . . 1 hr
    In class 0
    Eating and preparing for eating . . . . 1 hr
    Socializing . . . . 30 min
    Getting ready for bed, dressing, etc. 0
    Travel . . . . 1 hr 30 min
    Internet . . . . 2 hrs
  6 P.M. to bedtime
    Studying . . . . 30 min
    In class 0
    Eating and preparing for eating . . . . 1 hr
    Socializing . . . . 2 hrs
    Getting ready for bed, dressing, etc. 1 hr
    Travel 0
    Internet . . . . 1 hr

Now, complete an overall tally of the day's activities. How much time is spent on each general type of activity? Here is our example:

Hours spent on each type of activity
  Studying . . . . 2 hrs
  In class . . . . 1 hr
  Eating and preparing for eating . . . . 3 hrs

Socializing . . . . 2 hrs 30 min
Getting ready for bed, dressing, etc. . . . . 1 hr 30 min
Travel . . . . 1 hr 30 min
TV/Internet. . . . . 4 hrs

By examining this summary chart, one can consider whether they are spending too much or too little time in any activity. (Our student may be shocked to find that 4 hours are spent on watching TV and surfing the Net.) This can be enough to promote change. One can also identify warning cues for activities that are wasting time. Our student noted that he tended to waste time watching TV right after eating a meal or snack; eating was a cue.

SECTION 3: GOALS AND PRIORITIES

If one has difficulty determining how to allocate time, it can be useful to step back and examine long-term goals and priorities. What really matters? What will make someone truly happy when they retire? Different people have different values, including:

Adventure
Artistic creation and expression
Beauty
Discovery
Fame and recognition
Family
Financial success
Love
Personal effectiveness
Power
Spirituality and "meaning of life"

Next, what are one's lifetime goals and five-year objectives? What are one's objectives for the next 3–6 months? Examples of long-term, five-year, and six-month goals include:

Life-time goals
    To have children.
    To make enough money to be comfortable.
    To keep healthy.
Five-year goals
    To finish college.
    To get a meaningful job.
    To get married.

Six-month goals
  To manage stress better.
  To finish my second year of college.
  To move away from my family and live alone.
  To make the basketball team.
  To win at least one game of Monopoly with friends.

After considering goals, ask which are most and less important. Which need to be attended to today and which can be put off? Finally, break important immediate goals into concrete, specific, and realistic steps. Brainstorm possible courses of action, and review costs and benefits of the realistic choices. Our example student selected stress management, passing the science requirement, and deciding on a major as 6-month goals, with the following intermediate steps:

Managing stress better
  Read this book.
  Complete the exercises in this book.
  Practice relaxation exercises in this book.

Passing my science requirement
  Talk to others about science courses I could pass.
  Determine what science courses are important for my future.
  Which science courses are offered each semester?

Deciding on my major
  Talk to my advisor and parents.
  Look at job market.
  Look at courses I do best in.
  Go to career assessment office.

Once a client has decided upon immediate steps that have to be taken, short-term priorities for today and this week can be considered. Lakein suggests developing "top drawer," "middle drawer," "bottom drawer," and "wastebasket" priorities. Top drawer priorities are the most important tasks today and this week. The middle drawer includes activities that would be nice, but are not absolutely essential to do right away. Bottom drawer priorities are low-urgency activities that can be put off until top and middle drawer tasks are finished. Finally, "wastebasket" priorities include tasks that are a waste of time and do not have to be completed ever.

Our example person developed the following chart of priorities for this week:

Top Drawer
  Read chapter in stress management book. Practice exercises.
  Read the first two chapters in my Physics text.

Read the second chapter in my English text.
Ask John out for dinner.

Middle Drawer
Read ahead chapter 3 in Physics, if there is time.
Decide where I should spend my vacation.

Bottom Drawer
Watch TV.
Talk with friends.

Waste Basket
Snack.

Today's priorities include:

Top Drawer
Read chapter in stress management book. Practice exercises.
Read Chapter 1 in Physics text.
Phone up John.

Middle Drawer
Read English chapter

Bottom Drawer
Watch TV.
Talk with my friends (I can do that tomorrow).

Wustebasket
Snack.

SECTION 4: SCHEDULING

The goal of the preceding steps is to prepare for writing a schedule. Here one schedules activities for every half-hour period of time. Lakein suggests:

- Schedule in periodic times for reward and relaxation.
- Remember obligations over which you have no control.
- Pick the best time to do your important activities. Internal prime time is the best time for private or personal work, whereas external prime time is when external resources are most available.
- Schedule a reasonable period of time for each activity.

CONCLUSIONS

We conclude with a word of caution. Even the best of schedules is worthless if it is not put into action, or if it is derailed by distraction and diversion. We consider such impediments in the following chapter on procrastination.

EXERCISES

1. Complete a time-management schedule as outlined in this text. What were the most difficult parts of this chart to complete? Why?
2. If you were to implement your time management schedule (above), what are the most likely difficulties you might encounter? Think of two "backup strategies" (chapter 7) for dealing with each.
3. Consider the following distorted beliefs discussed in chapter 6: Fortune-Telling, Unrealistic Isolation, Childlike Fantasy, Helplessness, Mind-reading, and Minimizing. How might each contribute to problems with time management?
4. Think of effective counter statements for each of the above distorted beliefs that contributes to time management problems for you.

13

Procrastination

Procrastination is the avoidance of a task one has chosen to complete. Research (Ferrari, Johnson, & McCown, 1995) reveals two general patterns of procrastination, *anxious avoidance* and *lack of conscientiousness*. Anxious and avoidant individuals avoid tasks because of the fear and tension they arouse. Often they fear failure or perceive the procrastinated task as unpleasant or threatening. Lack of conscientiousness generally includes an absence of general work related skills, including time management problems, low motivation to complete a task, impulsiveness, and the tendency to focus on short-term rather than long-term rewards (doing things for the moment rather than delaying immediate gratification for a greater distant reward).

When a desired and chosen task is avoided, and simply not completed, one is deprived of the potential reward of success. What then maintains procrastinating behavior? Short-term payoffs include:

- The possibility a frustrating task or problem will be done or solved by someone else.
- By avoiding a task one avoids facing a feared failure.
- An avoided problem may resolve itself.
- The cost of completing a task in the future may be less (the "year-end sale" promise).
- By procrastinating one "gets even" or expresses passive-aggression to those expecting or demanding task completion.
- Procrastination may enable one to "cool off" and approach a threatening task more objectively.

Unfortunately, such rewards are often short-term and outweighed by longer-term negative consequences of avoiding an activity. Indeed, the fear of such a prospect may contribute to increased anxiety, which itself may increase one's tendency to procrastinate.

SECTION 1: TREATING PROCRASTINATION

Anxious avoidant procrastinators appear to benefit from procedures to reduce anxiety, and those displaying lack of conscientiousness benefit from treatments focusing on increasing concern, task-motivation, and thinking ahead (Ferrari, Johnson, & McCown, 1995).

Techniques for Both Anxious Avoidance and Lack of Conscientiousness

Problem-solving techniques are an important part of procrastination treatments. Specifically, one begins by identifying specific and concrete goals. Silver (1974) has suggested that procrastinators often perseverate on parts of a task they feel are easy (and put aside other parts). This can be countered by clearly articulating goals. Burns (1990) emphasizes making a job easy, either by breaking it down into logical steps or completing work in "small spurts." Here one commits to doing say fifteen or thirty minutes of a task (no more) a day, until it is done. The advantage of the small spurt approach is that it frees the procrastinator from worrying about how a task when viewed as a whole might be overwhelming.

Cognitive techniques form the heart of procrastination treatments for both anxious avoidant and unconscientious procrastinators. Typically one identifies, challenges, and changes distorted task-related thoughts that lead to task avoidance. Perhaps the simplest distortions are simple misperceptions about the amount of time or work required to complete a task (or the amount of time left before a deadline). A beginning college student may underestimate the time required to read a chapter, or the necessity of attending lectures in order to pass. These distortions are readily corrected through convincing information and explanation, either from supervisors and teachers, or from coworkers and classmates.

Ferrari, Johnson, and McCown (1995) suggest other forms of procrastination are associated with motivation-associated distortions, including:

- Overestimating future motivational states ("I'll feel like doing this later"),
- Assuming that success at a task requires one be in a positive task-oriented mood and "feel smart, energized, motivated, awake, and calm"; and
- Assuming that task failure or reduced productivity is the result of lack of such states.

Finally, most experts propose that procrastinators also harbor perfectionistic distortions, such as (Burka & Yuen, 1983):

- Assuming one must be perfect.
- Thinking everything one does should go easily and without effort.
- Believing that if it's not done right, it's not worth doing at all.
- Thinking that if one does well this time, one must *always* do well.
- Believing following someone else's rules means one is giving in and is not in control.
- Assuming there is one right answer, and one should wait until they find it.

Aaron Beck 1993) has a clever approach for dealing with distorted procrastination beliefs: the "TIC-TOC Technique" (Burns, 1990). Here a client identifies Task-Interfering Cognitions ("TICs") and then replacement thoughts, or Task-Oriented Cognitions ("TOCs"). For example, one might identify the following TIC:

"I shouldn't start unless I know exactly how everything will turn out."

This thought appears to be distorted, and fails the "reality check." Few of us know how all of our plans will turn out in the end, and often we have to settle for less than what we want. Such analysis could lead to this replacement TOC:

"I might as well start; I am sure I will at least get part of what I want."

Finally, relapse prevention (chapter 7) is a very useful general tool for treating procrastination. After a client has identified a desired goal, plan, and distorted, task-interfering cognitions, it is useful to consider how to counter relapse into procrastination. One general technique is identifying avoidant and distracting behaviors. What diversionary activities does the procrastinator engage in? What distorted beliefs and rationalizations does the procrastinator give for engaging in these activities rather than the chosen task? Knaus (1998), following Ellis's groundbreaking and somewhat rambling book on procrastination, places additional emphasis on such diversionary activities. Some activities, such as watching TV or reading the paper, can be easy to identify. Somewhat more complex is the self-induced conflict. Here one becomes preoccupied with a pseudoconflict that diverts one from a primary task. For example, the procrastinator may take time off to eat a snack, and then become preoccupied with conflicts about whether or not to actually consume a snack that might be fattening.

Anxious Avoidance

Given the role of anxiety in some forms of procrastination, it is reasonable that relaxation training should be a part of treatment. This is especially important when anxiety is so high as to be debilitating. Here, the full relaxation-training protocol presented in chapter 4 would be appropriate, incorporated into exposure or stress inoculation training (chapter 7). Specifically, one identifies the procrastinated task that evokes anxiety and pairs increasingly challenging versions with relaxation in stress inoculation training. I recommend stress inoculation training because of its focus on relapse prevention, which for the anxious avoidant individual would be a relapse into procrastinating thought and behavior.

For less debilitating anxiety that involves discomfort over avoidant tasks, I recommend relaxation techniques that appear to evoke relaxation-states associated with increased energy and alertness. These include breathing exercises and yoga stretching (chapter 4). Such techniques can be scheduled immediately prior to a procrastinated task. I would avoid techniques that can evoke disengagement, such as progressive muscle relaxation, autogenic training, and possibly imagery and meditation.

Lack of Conscientiousness

For procrastinators displaying lack of conscientiousness, Ferrari, Johnson, and McCown (1995) recommend less emphasis on relaxation and more on irrational beliefs regarding task completion. Morally-tinged scare tactics such as scolding, cajoling, or threatening are generally ineffective. Instead, it is more effective to take a nonjudgmental and practical approach, focusing on what goals one actually wants to complete and accurately estimating the amount of time and work needed to complete a task.

One clever challenge technique for those displaying lack of conscientiousness is to write down the amount of time one expects a task will take before starting work, and then record the actual time required. Often the discrepancy between estimated and actual time is a powerful motivator to examine distorted beliefs associated with procrastination. Another simple strategy for dealing with chronic underestimation of required time is to double the time one thinks it will take to finish a task.

SECTION 2: THE PROCRASTINATION PROTOCOL

Considering the ideas suggested in this chapter, I suggest a general treatment plan for treating procrastination, the *procrastination protocol*. Treatment includes the following steps.

1. *Complete procrastination inventory; Identify procrastinated task.* Here one either lists all of the times the previous week he or she has procrastinated, or plans to note during the subsequent week every time chosen tasks are put off. He or she then identifies a target procrastinating behavior for consideration. This is the task one will work on throughout the rest of the treatment protocol. Using the problem-defining techniques in

chapter 5, one clarifies if indeed the task goal is desired, how it can be broken into subgoals, and if perhaps a subgoal would be a more appropriate target procrastination task. Once a goal is identified, the costs and benefits of completing the goal are considered. If necessary, the task is revised.

2. *Identify avoidant behaviors.* One recalls, or records every day throughout the week, behaviors completed instead of the procrastinated task. These include activities that distract one from beginning a task as well as those that divert one from a course of action in midstream. The costs and benefits of avoidant behaviors are considered.

3. *Identify and remove cues for avoidant behaviors.* One examines environmental cues that may trigger or suggest avoidant behaviors (interesting magazines lying around, visible piles of snacks, fun-loving roommates or coworkers) and strategies for removing these cues. One considers aversive stimuli to follow avoidant strategies.

4. *Identify, challenge, and replace procrastinating distorted beliefs.* One then considers the main procrastinating distorted beliefs presented in this chapter and then thinks of personal examples of such distorted beliefs, perhaps including rationalizations for not including step 1 in this treatment protocol. Distorted beliefs that support both noncompletion of a desired task and completion of avoidant behaviors are considered. Each is disputed and countered (chapter 6) with a realistic task-oriented statement. Over the week one might spend a few minutes at the end of each day identifying and replacing procrastinating thoughts that arise.

5. *Complete stress inoculation training (for anxious avoiders).* Using the instructions in chapter 7, one creates a hierarchy of ten increasingly demanding versions of an avoided, anxiety-arousing task. Associated distorted beliefs and avoidant behaviors are reviewed. One then deliberately schedules two situations in which one relapses into procrastination after attempting to cope, and then deploys a comeback strategy. Each version is rehearsed in a relaxed state of mind until the entire sequence can be completed.

6. *Establish a task-conducive environment.* One identifies reminder-cues that enhance motivation and reinforce goal-directed behavior and supportive beliefs. Such cues can include posters, paper notes, work resources (dictionaries, phone books, computers). These are placed in one's task environment.

7. *Contract for completing the target task, create backup plan, complete task.* One then decides upon a time, place, and setting to complete the selected procrastinated task or task component. He or she decides ahead of time a self-given reward for successful completion. Part of the contract should include a backup plan for what to do if one procrastinates instead of completing the task. A useful backup plan might be to repeat protocol steps.

Illustration of the Procrastination Protocol

A student is having difficulty completing reading assignments for a class. He puts all reading off until the last week of class, and then crams for the final exam (which he usually fails). Here is how he proceeds with the suggested treatment protocol.

1. *Identify procrastinated task.* Obviously the desired task is reading the textbook before the final exam. This is too big a task to undertake at once, so it is broken down into components, reading one chapter a week. The costs of not completing this task include: increased anxiety about failing the exam, and lack of certainty about when one will actually do the work. Benefits of completing the task are: increased likelihood of passing the exam, improved self-esteem.

2. *Identify avoidant behaviors.* Instead of reading an assignment, the student generally goes to the student coffeehouse to meet and make new friends.

3. *Identify and remove cues for avoidant behaviors.* Our student usually phones his friends before going to a coffee house. He limits this cue by telling his friends ahead of time that he will not be available during his study time. In addition, he usually keeps a student newspaper on his desk, with advertisements announcing coffeehouse activities. He puts these papers away before studying.

4. *Identify, challenge, and replace procrastinating distorted beliefs.* Our student rationalizes that he can afford to put off reading the text and can read the text in one week before the exam. He checks how realistic this belief is by asking other students who have passed the exam when they have read the book, and discovers that most say that it is impossible to read the entire book before the exam. Another rationalization our student has is that somehow going to the coffeehouse will put him in such a good mood that he will want to study and will be able to study more effectively. After some thought, he realizes that he never studies after going to the coffeehouse, and that effective study does not require "getting into a good mood" first.

5. *Complete stress inoculation training (Not applicable for this student).*

6. *Establish a task-conducive environment.* The student makes some changes in his study nook. Study reminders, such as dictionaries and texts, are placed in view. Motivational statements countering distorted procrastinating behaviors are posted.

7. *Contract for completing the task, create backup plan, complete task.* Our student contracts to study from 7 to 9 p.m. every Wednesday evening. His reward will be to go to the student coffeehouse after studying. If he slips into a procrastinating pattern and fails to study, he contracts to spend one hour the next day reviewing: (1) whether or not he really

wants to pass the course (costs and benefits), (2) what additional avoidant behaviors (what goes on in the coffeehouse that diverts him from studying) interfere with the task, (3) additional distorted beliefs that support procrastination, and (4) what contract he will make. This new contract should be made with a friend or colleague, and both should agree that it is acceptable.

SECTION 3: DEALING WITH PROCRASTINATORS

It is hard enough to deal with procrastination in oneself. It can be even more difficult to deal with procrastination in others, especially when one has learned to view procrastination objectively as a habit rather than a moral flaw. Burka and Yuen (1983) have useful suggestions for coping with coworkers and classmates who procrastinate. Put briefly, they include:

1. Publicly establish clear limits, deadlines, and consequences—what has to be done when. Make sure they are mutually agreed upon.
2. Help the procrastinator establish small, manageable, interim goals.
3. Help the procrastinator be concrete and realistic about goals and tasks.
4. Reward interim progress. Specify exactly the behavior that is being rewarded and how it contributes to the long-term goal.
5. Be honest with your irritations and frustrations (perhaps using the DESC script in chapter 11).
6. Be clear in letting procrastinators know what you value in them. Which of their behaviors do you see as appropriate and effective? When do they actually engage in accurate reality-checking, problem-solving, and goal-defining?

SECTION 4: CONCLUSIONS

What can one do when one's best efforts to implement a stress management task fail? At one level, such a "failure" in itself becomes the problem (a relapse) calling for a renewed application of the tools of this book. However, when it becomes clear that a pattern of stress management setbacks is the result of ambivalence, lack of motivation, or self-sabotage, then it may be time to step back and review one's basic goals and values. This we consider in our final chapter.

EXERCISES

1. Complete the suggested Procrastination Protocol.
2. Consider the following distorted beliefs discussed in chapter 6: Fortune-Telling, Unrealistic Isolation, Childlike Fantasy, Helplessness, Mind-reading, and Minimizing. How might each contribute to problems with procrastination?
3. Think of effective counterstatements for each of the above distorted beliefs that contribute to procrastination for you.

14

Relaxation Beliefs, Active Coping Beliefs, and Philosophy of Life

We live in an age of threat and uncertainty. We live in uncentered times. In this concluding chapter we return to our first pillar of stress management—relaxation. Recall our definition: centering is relaxation. To be centered is to sustain passive simple focus; it is to *let go of needless distracting thought and tension and simply focus on the task, need, or want at hand.* This we do when we practice a formal relaxation discipline, one that truly fits our needs and beliefs. We also center when we solve the complexities of a problem, challenge distorted thinking, or calm the fire of a stressor through paced review or rehearsal. We center when we resolve interpersonal misunderstanding, miscommunication, and conflict. And we center when we pace our hectic lives and take action at the appropriate time. This has been a book on centering.

Returning to relaxation, research (Smith, 2001) clearly shows that one variable can profoundly deepen one's experience of centering—beliefs about why relaxation is important. Relaxation beliefs (R-Beliefs) significantly enhance the likelihood of experiencing a full range of positive states, extending from simple physical relaxation to feeling energized, joyful, loving, and even spiritual. And R-Beliefs provide an answer to the "why question" we encountered when discussing cognitive change (chapter 6). Why relax? Why experience deep relaxation-related states? The voices of over a thousand research participants suggest several answers:

Deeper Perspective (Life has a purpose greater than my personal wants and desires)

God (God guides, loves, and comforts me; I put myself in God's hands)

Inner Wisdom (I trust the body's wisdom and healing powers; there are sources of strength and healing deep within me)

Taking It Easy (Sometimes it is important to know when to stop trying, let go, and relax)

Acceptance (Sometimes it is important to accept things that cannot change)

Optimism (I believe in being optimistic, both in general and about how well I will deal with current hassles)

I suspect our beliefs also contribute to how effectively we actively cope with life's demands. Such beliefs provide an answer to the question "why is active coping important to me?" Although I have no research to offer, I propose a partial list of active coping beliefs:

It is important for me to get what I want without hurting others.

It is important for me to grow and fulfill my potential.

It is important for me to live a life in which I care for, teach, and inspire other people.

It is important for me to have good, open, and honest relationships.

It is important for me to experience and enjoy as much as I possibly can.

It is important for me to increase my strength, power, and knowledge.

It is important for me to create and appreciate beauty.

It is important for me to honor the best in my tradition.

It is important for me to learn as much as I can about myself and the world.

It is important for me to help serve society.

It is important for me to live long, healthily, and prosperously.

The value of articulating healthy active coping beliefs and R-Beliefs is that both provide a justification and motivation for pursuing stress management or relaxation outside of the practice session. ("It is important for me to live long and happily; I will try to be assertive whenever possible." "It is important for me to learn to let go when necessary; I will practice my yoga.") However, there is an important difference between the function of R-Beliefs and active coping beliefs.

PHILOSOPHIES OF RELAXATION: PHILOSOPHIES OF ACTIVE COPING

R-Beliefs provide the deepest reason one has for letting go of self-directed planful effort; active coping beliefs provide the deepest reason one has for pursuing centered, self-directed planful effort. In the world of relaxation, R-Beliefs reflect what I have (Smith, 1999a) termed the *paradox of passivity*. To elaborate, in everyday life discursive effort is required for success. Everything we do requires some form of planning and effort. Paradoxically, the opposite is true for relaxation. The less one actively plans a relaxation exercise, that is, how to do it, where it goes, feelings that should emerge, the better it works. Deliberately forcing a yoga stretch, breathing, or meditation will ruin the exercise; one has to focus and let go.

Effective R-Beliefs facilitate this paradoxical goal of trying and not trying by identifying, or acknowledging, that there is more going on than our everyday planful effort. Put differently, effective R-Beliefs suggest that the very direction and movement of a relaxation/centering exercise is not the result of our deliberate efforts and plans, but of some other "centering source." Some R-Beliefs are more or less explicit in naming this source (Deeper Perspective, God, Inner Wisdom). Others simply suggest that letting go opens doors (Acceptance, Taking it Easy).

In contrast, active coping beliefs typically point in what often seems to be a different direction, that ultimately one is personally responsible for one's fate, responsible for one's choices. For example:

> "I *want* to effectively define and solve problems." Why is that important for me? "So I *can* increase my knowledge and effectiveness."
>
> "I *want* to think more realistically." Why? "So I *can* live a more fulfilling life, and not be burdened with neurotic emotion."
>
> "I *want* to put into action my coping plans." Why? "So *I can* actually get what I *want* and not just dream about it."

In other words, the active techniques and strategies outlined in this book are ways of enhancing *personal efficacy*, a creative "I can do it" optimism.

PILLARS IN COLLISION? THE CHALLENGE OF RELAXATION AND CENTERING vs. ACTIVE COPING

A potential fundamental conflict, perhaps even a source of threat and uncertainty, exists between relaxation and the active pillars of stress management. Yes, at the practical level, relaxation is often incorporated into coping strategies. However, the potential for confusion exists. Our research has found that one of the most frequent barriers people have to learning relaxation is the distorted fear that such techniques will lead to withdrawal from active life. Our research (Smith, 2001) has identified what some such concerns are, as seen in Table 14.1.

As we have seen, there is indeed a difference between relaxation and active coping when we look at underlying supporting beliefs. Active coping beliefs help one be honest and true to oneself in a life of action; R-Beliefs help one be honest and true to what might be beyond oneself in the world of silence in relaxation. However, needless conflict and tension arise when R-Beliefs are pitted against active coping beliefs (for example,

**TABLE 14.1   Problems and Concerns People Most Often
                     Have with Relaxation**

Relaxation-induced anxiety
  I might become too sensitive to my problems when practicing relaxation.
  I might discover things I don't want to know.
  I might have strange (or uncomfortable) experiences.
  I might become more aware of my problems.
  I might lose touch with reality.

Unwanted disengagement
  Relaxation might slow me down too much.
  I might spend less times at things that are important.
  I might withdraw.
  Relaxation might interfere with coping and problem solving.
  I might become less effective (at work, school, sports, etc.) when relaxing.

Fantasy concerns
  Relaxation is too much like daydreaming.
  I might get lost in my fantasies while relaxing.

Trainer concerns
  I might get a relaxation trainer who does not tailor techniques for me.
  A trainer might not teach me what is best for me.

Practical concerns
  I might not slow down enough for relaxation to work.
  I might get distracted by other things while relaxing.
  I might find it hard to put relaxation to use in everyday life.

Religious/hypnotic control concerns
  Religious concerns might cause problems for me.
  I might become hypnotized in relaxation.

arguing that religious living is better than a life of social service; that self-less spirituality is better than self-affirming and shared pleasure; that work is better than play; making money is better than making music; wakefulness is better than sleep). In fact, quiet is just as important as action. And in centered action, both become one.

Let me conclude this book, not with another bullet list of options, but with a question, a challenge. Perhaps one of the most difficult tasks of stress management is to articulate a philosophy of life that includes both one's deepest reasons for experiencing the stillness of relaxation and centering, and one's deepest purpose for centered active living. Such a philosophy encompasses the entire rainbow and can serve as a true beacon in a world of threat and uncertainty.

Appendix

The Factor Structure of the Smith Irrational Beliefs Inventory—A

Julie D. Jenks

At least a half dozen inventories are available for assessing irrational beliefs (Robb & Ricks, 1990). All have relied on a trait or dispositional format in which respondents indicate how they "generally" or "typically" feel. The Smith Irrational Beliefs Inventory (SIBI) is the first test of irrational thinking that uses a situational format. Here irrational beliefs are rated as they pertain to a specific, client-selected stressful situation.

I administered the SIBI-Version A (see Table A.1) to 547 college students selected from six 4-year and junior colleges in the Chicago area and Iowa. All relevant APA guidelines were followed. The sample included 155 males, 375 females, and 17 undetermined (average age = 23.13 years, sd = 6.98).

A principal-components factor analysis with varimax rotation (the most frequently used approach in factor-analytic studies of irrational beliefs) yielded five factors with eigenvalues of at least 1.0 and with items loading at least .40 on only one factor (8 iterations). Then, a series of reliability analyses was performed on each factor, deleting items that did not contribute to reliability. Resulting factor scales (with item loadings) included:

Distorted Isolation: "Deep mistrust," .68; "Imperfections = unlovability," .65; "Unrealistic isolation," .64; "Rigid either/or thinking," .62; "Desperate need for love and caring," .58; "Emotion-distorted thinking," .43; Chronbach's alpha = .78, eigenvalue = 7.30, cumulative variance accounted for = 31.70 .

Catastrophizing and Fortune-telling "Fortune-telling," .77; "Possibilities = probabilities," .65; "Negative judgmental labeling," .64; "Negative spin," .59; "Ignoring contrary evidence," .54; "Catastrophizing," .47. Chronbach's alpha = .80, eigenvalue = 1.47, cumulative variance accounted for = 38.09.

Perfectionism: "Needless perfectionism," .77; "Musts/shoulds/oughts," .67; "Needless self-blaming," .48. Chronbach's alpha = .60, eigenvalue = 1.19, cumulative variance accounted for = 43.26.

Distorted Egocentrism "Special privilege," .77; "Needless other-blaming," .60; "Childlike fantasy," .56. Chronbach's alpha = .54, eignevalue = 1.13, cumulative variance accounted for = 51.80

Fatalistic Helplessness. "Helplessness," .71; "Fatalism and regretting the past," .43. Chronbach's alpha = .44, eigenvalue = 1.01, cumulative variance accounted for = 52.43.

TABLE A.1   Smith Irrational Beliefs Inventory—Version A

Nearly everyone experiences stress one time or another. Think of sometime over the past two weeks when you experienced a specific stressful situation or event (not "I'm always stressed out"). What were you doing? Where were you? Who was there? What did you want? What went wrong? In the box below, NAME THE STRESSFUL SITUATION OR EVENT you have in mind.

MY STRESSFUL SITUATION OR EVENT

Often our thoughts make stress worse. Below are some common types of unproductive and distorted stress-producing thinking. Please check how much you thought each in your stress situation (in the box above). Use this key:

IN THE ABOVE STRESS SITUATION OR EVENT . . .

① = I DIDN'T think this way at all
② = I thought this way A LITTLE
③ = I thought this way SOMEWHAT
④ = I thought this way A LOT.

---

① ② ③ ④   HELPLESSNESS: Believing you just can't cope by yourself and need much help and support from others. "I just deal with things by myself." "I always need help on important problems."

① ② ③ ④   CATASTROPHIZING. Turning simple frustrations, irritations, and disappointments into unbearable disasters and catastrophes. "I didn't get that raise (good grade, date, etc.); therefore it is the end of the world for me." "Things didn't turn out like I wanted; this is a disaster."

① ② ③ ④   DESPERATE NEED FOR LOVE AND CARING. Thinking that your need for love and caring are so important (or strong) that no one can or will ever meet them. "The kind of love I need no one can provide." "I am nothing without friends or lovers."

① ② ③ ④   NEGATIVE FORTUNE TELLING: Consistently predicting the future negatively, typically thinking that things will only get worse. "I'll fail that exam or won't get the job." "I will never be really contented."

① ② ③ ④   NEGATIVE JUDGMENTAL LABELING: Putting overall global negative labels on yourself or others. "I'm just a failure." or "He's a no good person."

① ② ③ ④   POSSIBILITIES = PROBABILITIES. Thinking that if it is possible for something to go wrong, then it is probable. "If I can mess up, I will." "If there's any chance things won't go my way, they won't."

TABLE A.1   Smith Irrational Beliefs Inventory—Version A *(Continued)*

① ② ③ ④   IGNORING CONTRARY EVIDENCE: Focusing on negative evidence while ignoring or discounting equally relevant positive evidence. "No one likes me. The fact that you like me doesn't count." "I'll never succeed. My college degree and job aren't important ."

① ② ③ ④   "MUSTS, OUGHTS, AND SHOULDS": Turning simple honest desires and wants into absolute musts, oughts, and shoulds. "I must be a success." (Rather than "It sure would be nice to be successful, but that may or may not happen.") Or: "I should be more likable (hard-working, relaxed, rich, religious, etc")." (Rather than "I would like to be more likable.")

① ② ③ ④   NEEDLESS SELF-BLAMING: Needlessly blaming yourself for negative events, and failing to see that some events have other, complex causes. "The only reason my marriage ended is because I failed." "I broke my leg because God is punishing me for my past sins."

① ② ③ ④   PREOCCUPATION ON REGRETTING THE PAST: Focusing on past wrongs, frustrations, and mistakes, rather than what you have or can do now. "So many things have gone wrong in my life." or "The past is filled with frustration."

① ② ③ ④   WHAT IF? WHAT IF? WHAT IF? Constantly asking "what if" something happens, and failing to be satisfied with any of the answers. "Yeah, but what if I get anxious?" or "What if I freeze up?"

① ② ③ ④   EMOTION -DISTORTED THINKING: Letting your feelings color and distort how you see the facts. "I feel depressed; therefore my marriage is not working out." "That person did something irritating, therefor I hate him. He's evil."

① ② ③ ④   NEEDLESS PERFECTIONISM: Picking an unfairly high standard for yourself and others, even though practically no one has ever been able to achieve it. "I should never do dumb things." "I have to be better than others."

① ② ③ ④   EXAGGERATING SIMPLE FEELINGS: Exaggerating simple, innocent emotions (that most people have) into terrible, overwhelming, psychiatric emergencies. "I must be depressed because I feel sad after my vacation." "It's dangerous to get nervous."

① ② ③ ④   SPECIAL PRIVILEGE: Claiming you have a special privilege or entitlement because you are somehow more important or deserving than others. "Everyone should always treat me nicely." "I should get what I want in life."

① ② ③ ④   RIGID, EITHER /OR THINKING: Viewing events or people in all-or-nothing terms and do not consider "shades of gray." "I get rejected by everyone," or "It was a complete waste of time."

TABLE A.1   *(Continued)*

① ② ③ ④	MIND-READING: Believing you know what others want, think, or feel without asking. "He doesn't like me. I just know it." "You're trying to analyze me. I can see it in your smile."
① ② ③ ④	NEEDLESS OTHER-BLAMING: Looking for someone else to blame when things don't go right. "My husband is to blame for the way I feel now," or "My mother caused all my problems."
① ② ③ ④	CHILDHOOD FANTASY: Assuming (as children may do) that everything should go your way. "Everyone should be nice and love each other." "Problems should have happy endings."
① ② ③ ④	MINIMIZING / AVOIDING: Understating or avoiding the true significance of events resulting in problems eventually becoming worse through inaction. "That problem's just in my mind." "I'll get over it."
① ② ③ ④	IMPERFECTIONS = UNLOVABILITY. Feeling that you are basically defective and flawed, making you unlovable to others if they find out."If people knew what I am really like, they would never like me." "I have flaws that will always keep people from accepting me."
① ② ③ ④	NEGATIVE SPIN. Arbitrarily and pessimistically putting a negative interpretation on events, even though they may be neutral or positive. "This is not what I really want." "I always look at the dark side of things."
① ② ③ ④	DEEP MISTRUST. Expecting that others willfully mistreat, dislike, manipulate, or take advantage of you. "Others are just out to get me." "You can't trust anyone."
① ② ③ ④	UNREALISTIC ISOLATION. Feeling that you are isolated from the rest of the world, different from other people, and are not, or cannot be part of any group or community. "I just don't belong." "I'm different from others."

NOTE: This version of the SIBI is presented for archival purposes. Those who desire to measure irrational beliefs should use the version presented in Table 6.1 (pp. 111–114).

References

Alberti, R. E. (1977). *Assertiveness: Innovations, applications, issues.* New York: Impact.

Alberti, R. E., & Emmons, M. L. (1982). *Your perfect right.* San Luis Obispo, CA: Impact.

American Psychiatric Association. (2000). *Diagnostic and statistical manual of mental disorders* (4th ed., text revision). Washington, DC: American Psychiatric Press.

Anderson, C. M., Reiss, D., & Hogarty, G. (1986). Family treatment of adult schizophrenic patients: A psychoeducational approach. *Schizophrenia Bulletin, 6,* 490–505.

Antony, M. M., & Swinson, R. P. (2000). *The shyness and social anxiety workbook.* Oakland, CA: New Harbinger.

Beck, A. T. (1976). *Cognitive therapy and the emotional disorders.* New York: International Universities Press.

Bedell, J. R., & Lennox, S. S. (1997). *Handbook for communication and problem-solving skills training: A cognitive-behavioral approach.* New York: Wiley.

Benson, H. (1975). *The relaxation response.* New York: Morrow.

Bohart, A. C., & Greenberg, L. S. (Eds.). (1997). *Empathy reconsidered: New directions in psychotherapy.* Washington, DC: American Psychological Association.

Borkovec, T. D. (1985). What's the use of worrying. *Psychology Today, 19,* 59–64.

Borkovec, T. D., Wilkinson, L., Folensbee, R., & Lerman, C. (1983). Stimulus control applications to the treatment of worry. *Behaviour Research and Therapy, 21,* 247–251.

Bower, S. A., & Bower, G. H. (1991). *Asserting yourself.* Cambridge, MA: Perseus Books.

Bryant, R. A., & Harvey, A. G. (2000). *Acute Stress Disorder.* Washington, DC: American Psychological Association.

Burka, J. B., & Yuen, L. M. (1983). *Procrastination: Why you do it and what to do about it.* Reading, PA: Addison-Wesley.

Burns, D. D. (1990). *The feeling good handbook.* New York: Plume.

Cannon, W. B. (1929). *Bodily changes in pain, hunger, fear, and rage.* New York: Appleton.

Caplan, G. (1964). *Principles of preventative psychiatry.* New York: Basic Books.

Cautela, J. R., & Wisocki, P. A. (1977). The thought-stopping procedure: Description, applications, and learning theory interpretations. *Psychological Record, 1,* 255–264.

Conger, J. C., & Farrell, A. D. (1981). Behavioral components of heterosocial skills. *Behavior Therapy, 12,* 41–55.

Curran, J. P., Wallander, J. L., & Farrell, A. D. (1985). Heterosocial skills training. In L. L'Abate & M. A. Milan (Eds.), *Handbook of social skills training and research* (pp. 136–169). New York: Wiley.

Davidson, R. J., & Schwartz, G. E. (1976). Psychobiology of relaxation and related states: A multiprocess theory. In D. I. Mostofsky (Ed.), *Behavior control and the modification of physiological activity* (pp. 399–422). Englewood Cliffs, NJ: Prentice-Hall.

Deffenbacher, J. L. (1999). Cognitive-behavioral conceptualization and treatment of anger. *Journal of Clinical Psychology, 55,* 295–309.

D'Zurilla, T. J., & Nezu, A. M. (1999). *Problem-solving therapy: A social competence approach to clinical intervention.* New York: Springer Publishing Co.

Egan, G. (1998). *The skilled helper* (6th edition). Pacific Grove, CA: Brooks/ Cole.

Ellis, A. (1962). *Reason and emotion in psychotherapy.* New York: Lyle Stuart.

Ellis, A. (1985). *Overcoming resistance: Rational-emotive therapy with difficult clients.* New York: Springer Publishing Co.

Ellis, A., & Dryden, W. (1997). *The practice of rational emotive behavior therapy.* New York: Springer Publishing Co.

Ferrari, J. R., Johnson, J. L., & McCown, W. G. (1995). *Procrastination and task avoidance: Theory, research, and treatment.* New York: Plenum.

Foa, E. B., & Kozak, M. J. (1986). Emotional processing of fear: Exposure to corrective information. *Psychological Bulletin, 99,* 20–35.

Friedman, M. J. (2000). *Post traumatic stress disorder.* Kansas City, MO: Compact Clinicals.

Gardner, M. (1957). *Fads and fallacies.* New York: Dover.

Gendlin, E. (1981). *Focusing.* New York: Bantam.

Goldstein, A. P., & Keller, H. (1987). *Aggressive behavior: Assessment and intervention.* New York: Pergamon Press.

Goldstein, A. P., & Rosenbaum, A. (1982). *Aggress-less.* Englewood Cliffs, NJ: Prentice Hall

Greenwald, H. (1973). *Direct decision therapy.* San Diego, CA: EDITS.

Greenwald, D. P. (1977). The behavioral assessment of differences in social skill and social anxiety in female college students. *Behavior Therapy, 8,* 925–937.

Gruen, R. J., Folkman, S., & Lazarus, R. S. (1988). Centrality and individual differences in the meaning of daily hassles. *Journal of Personality, 56,* 743–762.

Holmes, T. H., & Rahe, R. H. (1967). The social readjustment rating scale. *Journal of Psychosomatic Research, 11,* 213–218.

Hope, D. A., Heimberg, R. G., Juster, H. R., & Turk, C. L. (2000). *Managing social anxiety: A cognitive-behavioral therapy approach.* San Antonio, TX: The Psychological Corporation.

Horowitz, M. J. (1982). Psychological processes induced by illness, injury, and loss. In T. Millon, C. Green, & R. Meagher (Eds.), *Handbook of clinical health psychology* (pp. 53–67). New York: Plenum.

Ivey, A. E., Ivey, M. B., & Simek-Morgan, L. (1997). *Counseling and psychotherapy: A multicultural perspective* (4th ed.) Needham Heights, MA: Allyn & Bacon.

Jacobson, E. (1929). *Progressive relaxation.* Chicago: University of Chicago Press.

Jakubowski, P., & Lange, A. J. (1978). *The assertive option.* Champaign, IL: Research Press.

Kleinke, C. L., Meeker, F. B., & Staneski, R. A. (1986). Preferences for opening lines: Comparing ratings by men and women. *Sex Roles, 15,* 585–600.

Knaus, W. J. (1998). *Do it now.* New York: Wiley.

Kukpke, T. E., Calhoun, K. S., & Hobbs, S. A. (1979). Selection of heterosocial skills, II. Experimental validity. *Behavior Therapy, 10,* 336–346.

Lakein, A. (1973). *How to get control of your time and your life.* New York: Signet.

Lazarus, R. S., & Folkman, S. (1984). *Stress, appraisal, and coping.* New York: Springer Publishing Co.

Leahy, R. L., & Holland, S. J. (2000). *Treatment plans and interventions for depression and anxiety disorders.* New York: Guilford Press.

Linden, W. (1990). *Autogenic training: A clinical guide.* New York: Guilford Press.

Linden, W. (1993). The autogenic training method of J. H. Schultz. In P. M. Lehrer & R. L. Woolfolk (Eds.), *Principles and practice of stress management* (pp. 205–229). New York: Guilford Press.

Luthe, W. (Ed.). (1969–1973). *Autogenic therapy* (Vols. 1–6). New York: Grune & Stratton.

Macan, T. H. (1994). Time management: Test of a process model. *Journal of Applied Psychology, 79,* 381–391.

Marlatt, A., & Gordon, J. (1984). *Relapse prevention: A self-control strategy for the maintenance of behavior change.* New York: Guilford Press.

McKay, M., Davis, M., & Fanning, P. (1995). *Messages: The communication skills book, second edition.* Oakland, CA: New Harbinger Publications.

McMullin, R. E. (2000). *The NEW handbook of cognitive therapy techniques.* New York: Norton.

Meichenbaum, D. (1985). *Stress inoculation training.* New York: Pergamon.

Mitchell, J. (1983). When disaster strikes . . . The critical incident stress debriefing process. *Journal of Emergency Medical Services, 8,* 36–39.

Mullin, R. E. (2000). *The NEW handbook of cognitive behavior therapies.* New York: Norton.

Novaco, R. (1975). *Anger control: The development and evaluation of an experimental treatment.* Lexington, MA: D. C. Heath.

Paul, G. L. (1966). *Insight versus desensitization in psychotherapy: An experiment in anxiety reduction.* Stanford, CA: Stanford University Press.

Peterson, R. J. (2000). *The assertiveness workbook.* New York: New Harbinger.

Plutchik, R. (1994). *The psychology and biology of emotion.* New York: HarperCollins.

Robb, H. B., & Ricks, W. (1990). Irrational belief tests: New insights, new directions. *Journal of Cognitive Psychotherapy, 4,* , 303–311.

Rubinstein, J. S., Meyer, D. E., & Evans, J. E. (2001). Executive control of cognitive processes in task switching. *Journal of Experimental Psychology—Human Perception and Performance, 4,* 763–797.

Russell, R. K., & Matthews, C. O. (1975). Cue-controlled relaxation in *in vivo* desensitization of a snake phobia. *Journal of Behavior Therapy and Experimental Psychiatry, 6,* 49–51.

Schiraldi, G. R. (2000). *The post-traumatic stress disorder sourcebook.* Los Angeles: Lowell House.

Schultz, J. H., & Luthe, W. (1959). *Autogenic training: A psychophysiologic approach in psychotherapy.* Stuttgart, Germany: Georg Thieme.

Selye, H. (1956). *The stress of life.* New York: McGraw-Hill.

Silver, M. (1974). Procrastination. *Centerpoint, 1,* 49–54.

Slaikeu, K. A. (1990). *Crisis intervention: A handbook for practice and research* (2nd ed.). Boston: Allyn and Bacon.

Smith, J. C. (1993a). *Creative stress management.* Englewood Cliffs, NJ: Prentice-Hall.

Smith, J. C. (1993b). *Understanding stress and coping.* New York: Macmillan.

Smith, J. C. (1999a). *ABC Relaxation Theory: An evidenced-based approach.* New York: Springer Publishing Co.

Smith, J. C. (1999b). *ABC Relaxation Training: A practical guide for health professionals.* New York: Springer Publishing Co.

Smith, J. C. (2001). *Advances in ABC Relaxation: Applications and inventories.* New York: Springer Publishing Co.

Smith, J. C., & Jackson, L. (2001). Breathing exercises and relaxation states. In J. C. Smith (Ed.), *Advances in ABC relaxation training: Applications and inventories* (pp. 190–192). New York: Springer Publishing Co.

Thoits, P. A. (1983). Dimensions of life events that influence psychological distress: An evaluation and synthesis of the literature. In H. B. Kaplan (Ed.), *Psychosocial stress* (pp. 33–103). New York: Academic Press.

Watson, J. C. (2002). Re-visioning empathy. In D. J. Cain & J. Seeman (Eds.), *Humanistic psychotherapies: Handbook of research and practice* (pp. 445–471). Washington, DC: American Psychological Association.

Wolpe, J. (1959). *Psychotherapy by reciprocal inhibition.* Stanford, CA: Stanford University Press.

Index